...ING LONELINESS AND MAKING FRIENDS

...IANNA CSÓTI taught at secondary level in the ...don Borough of Brent and was a houseparent at an ...ternational sixth-form college in South Wales for six years. She has written several books, including *Social Awareness Skills for Children*, *Contentious Issues: Discussion Stories for Young People* and *School Phobia, Panic Attacks and Anxiety in Children*. Her website is www.mariannacsoti.co.uk.

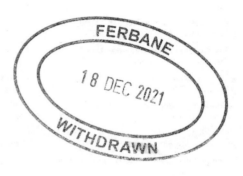

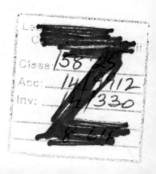

Overcoming Common Problems Series

Selected titles
A full list of titles is available from Sheldon Press,
36 Causton Street, London SW1P 4ST, and on our website at
www.sheldonpress.co.uk

Overcoming Common Problems Series

Overcoming Common Problems Series

Overcoming Common Problems

Overcoming Loneliness and Making Friends

Márianna Csóti

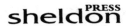

First published in Great Britain in 2005
Sheldon Press
36 Causton Street
London SW1P 4ST

The author and publisher have made every effort to
ensure that the external website addresses included
in this book are correct and up to date at the time of going
to press. The author and publisher are not responsible for the
content, quality or continuing accessibility of the sites.

British Library Cataloguing-in-Publication Data

A catalogue record for this book is available from the British Library

ISBN 0–85969–959–5

3 5 7 9 10 8 6 4 2

Typeset by Deltatype Limited, Birkenhead, Merseyside
Printed in Great Britain by
Ashford Colour Press

For my very dear friends

Contents

Introduction

Good friendships help us through the trials of life and provide company and entertainment. However, many people need help in either forming new friendships or in enhancing existing friendships. This may be because they are too shy, are lacking in social skills, or have other difficulties that interfere with forming satisfying and rewarding relationships. All these factors contribute to loneliness.

Some people associate loneliness with weird people who are best avoided. This is simply not true! Everyone experiences loneliness at some time in their lives, no matter what their age or sex: it is not confined to any one group of people, nor is it anything to feel ashamed about. The good thing is that loneliness does not have to be with you for life. There is something that can be done about it. We owe it to ourselves to change our lives for the better and reach out to other people, many of whom will also be experiencing loneliness.

1

Defining a friend

Friends are the spices and herbs of your life, adding colour and flavour to an otherwise bland existence; they are companions that help you live your life to the full. A mix of personalities and backgrounds in your friends allows for variation in what you talk about with them, what you do with them and how you do things with them.

Having good friends, where you have a high level of intimacy, sharing confidences and expressing feelings and opinions, is essential to being happy and emotionally healthy. And the depth of your friendships, or the level of intimacy that is between you and another person, is more important than the actual number of friends you have.

What friendships can mean to different people

Christian's friends are people with whom he goes to football and rugby matches, watches sport on television and plays five-a-side football after work. They are also his drinking companions in the pub. With his friends he talks about work, sport, holidays and school experiences.

Theresa's friends are shopping, cinema and clubbing companions. She also spends a great deal of time talking and listening to them. Since she has always lived in the same area she has kept up with her school friends. She found them especially helpful and supportive when her father died. When good things happen in any of the friends' lives, they all go out together to celebrate. Theresa's friendships with people at work are more casual and she only occasionally joins them for a drink at lunchtime or after work, when it is someone's birthday.

Marjorie's friends are people she sees at church and at Women's Institute functions. She also goes on courses with them. She gave much support to one of her friends after she was diagnosed with cancer.

Diane's friendships revolve around her children and she gets together with other women so that her children can play with their children. Sometimes she and her husband share their friends by having dinner parties. None of these friends are particularly close to Diane and she regrets having given up work, where her friendships were based more on personality similarities, rather than what ages mothers' children are.

Phil goes to clubs with his male friends who are mainly gay like him and has long chats with female friends from work.

From the above, it is clear that friends fulfil certain functions. For many, they are people to do things with such as play sport, go shopping or go on courses. These serve to fulfil the social role of friends. Sharing feelings, successes and disappointments through conversation and practical support serves to fulfil the emotional role of friends.

It tends to be more common for male friends to meet up to do things together rather than just talk – whereas meeting for a chat tends to be more common for women. Although men meet to chat in the pub, say, it is still less usual for their conversations to follow an intimate line, whereas women's conversations tend to be more intimate and may include analyses of relationships with other people, especially partners.

Having friends is also about fitting in. Phil's male friends are mainly gay. This may be because he has been socially, rather than sexually, rejected by many heterosexual men or because he likes to be with others who are like him to give him a sense of belonging. Of course, you can feel that you belong while celebrating your differences, but for this to work you need to rely on other people embracing those differences and accepting you for yourself. (See Chapter 7 for help on dealing with prejudices and stereotypes.)

Some friendships are born, and survive, through lifestyle similarities or mutual convenience. Marjorie's friends in the Women's Institute, for example, have time on their hands and need to find other people who have time on their hands. But they also have other things in common – they have all retired, are of a similar age and have few family commitments.

You might have a set of 'ready made' friends, who include you in activities just because you are there. People who live on an RAF base, for example, can conveniently socialize with others who live on the base – indeed, there are often social clubs on site to encourage this. The physical proximity between you and the other people, and the frequency of meeting, can provide you with the opportunity to develop intimate lifelong friendships.

New mothers at home with babies often find it convenient to get together with other new mothers, as friends from work or school are usually employed in the daytime; they can also share concerns about childcare and exchange information.

Friends also fulfil more than just your immediate needs. For example, Diane's friends are mainly those with children, so that her own children have others to play with on a regular basis.

Sometimes friendships can develop because of the need to live harmoniously. Going back to our example of an RAF base, you would need to be very careful about making disparaging remarks about other people from the base since it may get back to them. Having favourites or being too cliquey may lead to others feeling excluded, which in turn could build resentment and hurt – probably not a good idea in such a closed environment.

The length of friendships

This can vary, from a few days to for ever. Some friendships, once made, are made for life. They might be grounded in some common intense experience, which brought you close to someone else so that you might feel forever bound to that person regardless of the passing of the years or physical distance. You might, for example, both have been refugees living at the same camp, transported to the same host country and given work with the same employer. This common experience may have made it important for you both to keep in touch throughout your lives, no matter where you finally settled. Or perhaps a stranger saved the life of your only child and you feel forever indebted to that person. Or you might both have been in the same rail accident and suffered similar injuries.

These kinds of examples tend to be uncommon. More usually, life friendships can continue for more mundane reasons – you may continue to be close to a friend who shared your dormitory at boarding school, for example; or because you went to school in the area that you have lived in all your life, there is no need to make new friends, or at least break with the old ones.

Some friendships last for long periods, but not a lifetime. For example, if you made friends in an area in which you lived for ten years you may, on moving, devote your energies to making new friends. Or you may have made friends through work, but on changing jobs find there is not the motivation to continue the old friendships.

Some friendships last a very short time. For example, if you are on a five-day course, you may find you have paired up with another person, or have formed a group of friends who help each other with the assignments and share lunch and dinner breaks. But when the course ends you all go your separate ways without any firm commitment to meeting up again.

Social networks

Any friends that you have make up your social network. To map out your own social network, get a large sheet of paper and draw a small circle in the centre that represents you. Then draw circles on the page around you to represent your school friends, putting their initials in the centre. Connect their circles to yours using straight lines. If they socialize with each other as well, connect their circles too. Add circles to represent friends from work and indicate whether they socialize with each other by making further connections.

Likewise, draw in friends that socialize with you but no one else from your social network – I call them isolates. They should have only one line joining them to you.

You can now see how many friends you have at a glance. You will also see that those friends who socialize with other friends of yours form a clique. You might have one clique in your social network comprised of school friends, and another compromised of work friends. Or it may be that you have changed jobs and have cliques from different workplaces.

The advantage of a clique is that when something goes wrong in your life and you tell one of the other members, they will all support you, especially if it is to do with something that they can all understand such as a problem at work. One disadvantage of a clique is that if there is something very private you only want one other person to know, it is unlikely to be kept confidential. The temptation to tell another clique member might be too great, especially if it is a close-knit clique that meets frequently: soon all might know. Another disadvantage of a close-knit clique is that skills and knowledge within the group may be very similar (such as a lawyer having only friends connected through legal work): having a loose social network allows for larger variation in friends who are a part of other social networks. This also gives a greater possibility of having a friend who knows someone with expertise in other areas should you need it.

With a looser clique, there is obviously less intimacy, such as with old school friends who don't often meet up, or with a group who are all new to the same place of work. This kind of situation allows for the possibility for pairs or trios of very close friends within that loose clique, without necessarily compromising a need for confidentiality with the rest of the clique.

The advantage of having some friends that are isolates – that is, not socializing with anyone else who knows you – means that whatever you tell is likely to be kept confidential, as even if one of these friends does divulge what you say to someone else, it is not going to get back to the others in your social network. This type of friendship is great for those who have trouble in disclosing (see Chapter 5). If you have several isolates as friends, you can even disclose different things to different people to get the support you need, without anyone knowing the whole you – though you should try to aim for that with the most special person in your life. Ideally, to get the best of all types of friendship, you should try to have a mix of close-knit and loose cliques and isolates.

Social dissatisfaction

We all have our own desires for what we need in the way of friends. What might constitute a satisfying social network for one person may not for another, and if you feel that you must have a high number of friends, it is harder to be satisfied.

If you feel the need for more friends, add circles to your social network in a different colour to represent people you only know vaguely such as neighbours and people you know to say hello to (at your evening class, for example). Then decide which ones you might try to spend longer talking with, to see if you like each other, and whether both of you might want to get to know each other better – in other words, whether there is friendship potential here. It is often easier to make new friends this way than to try with a complete stranger.

Try to acknowledge that if you do have a fair number of friends, you don't necessarily need more to make you less lonely and, if you think you do, do you realistically have the time to keep these relationships going at the same level while making new friends? It might be more intimacy that you need. Or it might be that you want one special person with whom to share your life. In identifying where there is a genuine emotional need in yourself, you are more likely to be able to achieve your personal goal of a satisfying social network.

Making new friends

New friends can be made anywhere. Here are some of the places I've made friends: in school, in university, in hospital, in a soft play area in a leisure centre where I took my daughter, in my local gym, in my husband's workplace, in my workplaces in my role as a houseparent and in my role as a teacher, in the area in which I live (a college campus), and in my house when I have had someone help me with either childcare or cleaning. I have also made friends with parents of my daughter's friends and from someone I have contacted through the contacts page in a specialist magazine.

When I am out I enjoy chatting to taxi drivers, people that sit with me in waiting rooms or on a train, people in supermarkets and people I meet when I walk around the campus where I live. I am happy to say that my friends have little in common other than my liking and respecting them. They do not all share the same backgrounds, education, culture, or marital or employment status – but they do all share a love of humour.

Everywhere you go there is potential for social interaction, and without socially interacting with others you will never know whether there is also potential for friendship. If, however, you find it hard to hold prolonged conversations with strangers, try to meet people in an environment where you have something in common and where you are likely to be with that person for a longer time than when passing someone in the street.

You could join an evening class, either to learn more about a particular skill or for keeping fit, or a rambling group, or you could do voluntary work such as helping out in your religious community, a charity shop or becoming involved in conservation. You could attend a concert or go to the theatre and chat to the person sitting next to you. You could go to art galleries or museums and discuss what you see with someone else that is looking interested. If you have a young child you could go to the local park and talk to other parents of young children.

The course of friendship

When you first meet someone new, you have no idea whether that person will ever become a friend. This first meeting gives you a chance to find out a little about each other's background, education, hobbies, work, family, and so on. If you then feel you do have things in common, and would like to know the other person better, you might want to meet up again. This can be done much more easily and naturally if you are in a situation where you can meet without a formal arrangement, such as at an evening class or mothers and toddlers' group. This takes the pressure off and gives you the chance to continue getting to know someone within a clear social structure, until you feel ready to take the plunge and invite someone for coffee, or to meet up in the park with her children.

Of course, a first meeting can also rule out potential friendship 'candidates' if you feel you have nothing in common with the other person. Another preventative factor may be the distance involved between your respective homes, or their lifestyle factors such as simply being too busy with work and family.

If you do meet up again by design, or accident, and get on well, you will arrange subsequent meetings to find out more about each other. This period determines whether you will become close and firm friends, casual friends that meet up only occasionally or whether the burgeoning relationship dies altogether.

Some friendships are light and casual and will not progress to intimacy: this might be because neither party is prepared to confide in the other or because they have problems expressing their feelings and opinions and so prevent the other getting to know them closely. Or it might be because one of you has divulged something that makes the other feel uneasy or disapproving. Or it might be that the other person broke your confidence and you no longer trust him or her. In this case, you and your potential friend both need to choose whether to continue the relationship at that level or to put an end to the friendship. If the friendship continues, it doesn't always mean it will never move on to intimacy. But until the worrying thing is resolved or the person is tested with another confidence and pulls through, it is unlikely.

In friendships that do progress to intimacy both parties have high disclosures, where they confide deep emotions and disturbing events, and very much trust each other (see Chapter 5). If you are afraid of confiding and having your trust broken, you can minimize the risks by starting new relationships very slowly and taking each progressive step carefully. You can test the water by telling the other person tiny confidences about yourself, and wait to see if that makes a difference to how they view you and whether these confidences are broken because they are told to other people.

When you are sure of the ground and the other person has shared confidences back, you may then feel able to go a little deeper. The progression of the relationship can be halted at any time. It can even go backwards where there is less frequent contact and less sharing of confidences. However, if you do this with all your relationships, you won't find them particularly rewarding nor will you get much emotional support and others will see you as distant and uninvolved.

2

What is loneliness?

Loneliness is unhappy solitude: being socially apart from other people at a time when we want to feel included and feeling emotionally isolated, having no one with whom to share our inner thoughts, fears and dreams. It is possible to be lonely even if we are surrounded by people.

Loneliness is an important life issue to tackle. People that are lonely have poorer physical health. It is well known that sick people recover more quickly when they have someone to care for and care about them, even if it is a pet.

Being lonely and not having satisfactory relationships also adversely affects our mental health. It damages our self-esteem, the way we think and feel about ourselves, and our self-confidence. In severe and persistent loneliness, we may give up trying to make friends or relate to others, believing that 'there is no point as it never works out', which can lead to depression. Feeling lonely, together with the experience of social isolation, can make existing depression worse. Having someone to talk to, to share the ups and downs of our day and to have fun with is vitally important to feeling included and valued.

Types of loneliness

Emotional loneliness is about not having satisfying intimate friend-ships: not having someone to care about you or listen to your troubles. Or it may be that you are looking for someone special with whom to share your life. An emotionally lonely person may have a few friends, but the friendships are lacking in some way: perhaps feelings aren't shared or understood. When this happens you can feel empty, abandoned, worried and frightened.

Social loneliness is when you don't have friends to do things with or be with and you feel bored and marginalized, not being involved in what's going on. If, for example, you move to a new area or work shifts or work unsociable hours you may feel socially isolated.

Some people socially isolate themselves because they have too many rules about with whom they should mix. For example, if you believe that you should only talk to people of the same race, culture, religion, sexual orientation, class, etc. as you then you are limiting the number of possible social contacts you can make. You limit them further by avoiding people with disabilities, that don't look attractive, who aren't popular, are too old, too young, too thin, too fat ... Ask yourself if you have done this and, if so, ask yourself why you have written these people off as possible friends and if your reasons are valid. How would you feel if someone told you that you didn't fit into her ideas of the type of person she should befriend?

Loneliness can be acute and temporary such as when a young person starts university and doesn't know anyone else: it takes time to get to know people and make new friends. (See below and Chapter 9.)

Loneliness can be long-term and is more of a problem since a chronically lonely person is unhappy for a protracted period of time increasing the risk of depression and suicide.

Long-term loneliness prevents us from going out and doing positive things with our lives. We are more likely to remain at home doing something passive like reading, watching television, playing on the computer, spending time on the Internet and sleeping more than we need. We might turn to shopping, eating, alcohol or drugs to dull the emotional pain of loneliness and to help us sleep.

Some people try to prove to themselves and others that they are 'doing all right' by becoming very busy. This might be with hobbies, exercise or voluntary work. Or they may become workaholics. They may try to assuage their loneliness by joining chat rooms. (Also see 'Loneliness' in Chapter 3.)

The individuality of loneliness

Everyone's threshold for feeling lonely, and the circumstances in which they feel lonely, is different and individual to them. In the following scenarios, can you tell which people are lonely?

- Harold is an elderly bachelor who has lived alone all his adult life.
- May is an attractive, fun-loving 18-year-old girl at university for the first time.
- Aran is in his 30s, is married with children and has been in the same job for the past seven years.

- Preeti is 40, childless, and has just separated from her husband.
- Sean is 25 and has just moved into his first place having lived at home with his eight brothers and sisters all his life.

All of the above people could be lonely. However, although Harold is lonely he copes very well with his solitude as he has lived with it for so long, whereas May feels excruciatingly lonely and does not know how to deal with it. Aran, you might think, oughtn't to be lonely as he has so much in his life, but he is. He feels that intimacy is missing in both his marriage and with his friends.

Although Preeti feels devastated that her marriage has failed and that she now lives alone, she is actually relieved to be spared living with someone who was causing her loneliness as her husband's presence prevented her from meeting new people and moving on.

Despite living on his own after a life surrounded by so many siblings, Sean is thankful to have his own private and peaceful space. Sacrificing familial company was the price Sean had to pay for his longed-for independence, but he fills the void with his friends and by living his life how he wants to.

It isn't possible to label someone as lonely just by looking at his or her life. Although all of the above people have some sort of loneliness, it is only a big problem to May and Aran. The others are coping well with their lives and, apart from Harold, are confident that their loneliness is only temporary.

Variations in loneliness

How we perceive our needs for assuaging loneliness can vary over time. There may be periods in our life when we are quite satisfied with what we have until something happens that increases our need for intimacy such as bereavement, the loss of a job or another disappointment.

If, however, things are going well for us, we might not be prepared to make the time to maintain the intimacy of the relationships we do have, as we are so taken up with our own immediate lives. For example, if you are involved with a large project at work and the time you use overspills into your private life, you may so enjoy the challenge of creating or developing something new that you find it a nuisance to have to make time to see people.

The way you feel about yourself can also vary. Some days you might feel quite confident and happy with yourself and so not feel as great a need for social contact as the days when you are feeling less worthy and less assured of yourself.

Sometimes it is the days of the week that can make you feel lonely. If you are at work, weekdays may be quite sociable so when the weekend arrives you might feel lonely, especially if you live alone. If you are a parent at home with a young child you may feel less lonely at weekends when you have your partner to share your days.

Young, single people can feel much lonelier at weekends not necessarily because they are on their own more than in the week, but because they imagine everyone else their age has a better social life at weekends than they do. For example, staying in on a Friday or Saturday night is more painful to them than staying in on a weekday.

When you take annual leave you might feel lonelier if you have to go on holiday on your own or spend it in solitude at home, preferring the social contact of the workplace.

Enjoying solitude

If you spend several hours alone each day you may feel terribly lonely, but someone else in the same circumstances may not be lonely at all. Some people feel they are lonely when spending even short periods of time on their own, having a high need for interaction with other people and believing that if they are not with someone all the time, they must be lonely.

But some people enjoy being by themselves and need more time alone than other people. Indeed, they can become stressed if they don't get sufficient time to themselves. This might be a personality trait or it might be for other reasons, some of which are given below.

Some professions demand that a great deal of time is spent alone as this is necessary to get the work done. For example, if writers or artists are continually interrupted they are prevented from being immersed in their subject and the creative train of thought is broken; and religious people need time to reflect on their lives and to pray.

With some medical conditions, such as Asperger Syndrome on the autism spectrum, people will become stressed if they cannot be by themselves for a good part of their day, or when they feel the need to be alone.

Some only children may have become used to a quiet home atmosphere and have learnt to amuse themselves – and so find it daunting when in enforced and prolonged company of others; they may be relieved to be alone again.

So being alone does not always mean that someone is lonely. Our individual needs dictate whether we are lonely and, as with the variation in the number of friends different people need to satisfy them, the length of time socializing to satisfy them also varies.

However, friendship skills are good for everyone to learn, even the naturally solitary. There may come a time when you want to increase your social contact – or you may be required to work in a team in your occupation. It is also essential to have the skills to get on with people, not to give offence: even to tell them that you need more time to yourself.

Perception of loneliness

How we perceive loneliness and how we feel about it, and what expectations we have of our social life, can affect how lonely we feel.

Lonely people do not necessarily have fewer friends or social interactions than people who are not lonely, but they are more dissatisfied with what they do have. They may want more friends, or want more intimacy with the friends they have. Or they may want a special friend with whom to share their life, such as a long-term partner.

Loneliness is not an absolutely definable state: there is no fixed number of friends you should have in order to keep loneliness at bay. For example, just because we don't have the five close friends our work colleague does, it does not necessarily follow that we are lonely – or that she is not lonely. She could still be lonely with the five close friends, feeling the need for more. Another colleague might only have one close friend and not feel lonely at all.

The way we feel about being lonely affects our ability to cope with loneliness. One person may be very concerned that he is lonely, feeling desperate to change things whereas another may note the fact she is lonely but shrug it off in the belief that the situation is not serious and is not likely to last.

Another person may feel that being lonely is something to be ashamed of and try to hide the fact that he is lonely at all costs. Another may freely admit to it, especially if she feels her loneliness is understandable under the circumstances, such as a mother whose children are now all at school for the first time and whose days are completely free.

As well as having certain expectations about the number of friends we ought to have, we have expectations about how deep our relationships have to be to assuage our loneliness. Some people are fine with very superficial relationships whereas others desperately want someone with whom to share their everyday actions and thoughts, and someone to know and know them back intimately.

Gender and loneliness

Women often appear to experience loneliness more than men do, because of their liking and need for intimate conversations. Although men seem to avoid intimacy with other men, a woman friend can be valuable for allowing a man to open up without fearing loss of face or showing vulnerability.

There has been evidence to show (Howells 1981) that persistently lonely men are more likely to be aggressive and hostile towards other people, particularly women, and the lonelier and more isolated they become, the greater their aggression and hostility.

Loneliness and self-esteem

When we feel lonely our self-esteem can suffer, particularly if that loneliness is experienced long-term. We start to think we are no good, that no one likes us or loves us or that we are boring and not worth anyone's time and consideration. So feeling lonely is bad for our mental health. A shift in our personal belief system will help to prevent damage to our self-esteem.

If we believe that it is OK to occasionally feel lonely, and that lonely people are not worthless people we might feel better about ourselves. If we believe that it is OK to be on our own for some of the time and that to turn up to social events on our own is also OK we will feel better about ourselves.

It also helps to consider whether labelling ourselves as lonely has something to do with how we imagine other people's lives to be. Are we truly lonely or are we worrying that other people are labelling us as lonely? Or are we comparing the number of friends we have to the number of friends we think, or know that, other people have?

Sometimes it can help just to know that being alone does not necessarily make someone lonely. Being alone is not something to be ashamed of and therefore not something that should necessarily lower your self-esteem: there is no need to avoid social contact because you fear others will see you as lonely and therefore not worthy of getting to know. If you did, avoidance of social contact would ensure you remained lonely in the long term.

If, for example, you were at a party and saw someone arrive unaccompanied but smiling and friendly to the people there, you would not label her as lonely. So there is no need to fear that anyone would label you as lonely on the sole fact that you are on your own at a social event. If you feel that wherever you go it is obvious that you are a lonely person, adjusting your behaviour on the advice given in this book will help change that.

Gail

Gail felt she was lonely. She didn't work because of health problems, her children were all old enough to attend school and her husband worked long hours and was often away from home. Although she saw friends, they were often busier than she, so her social contact was limited by their lifestyles rather than her own. She spent much time on the Internet emailing friends from before her marriage and move to another town, and others that lived close by but had time pressures. Gail felt she lacked close friends.

When Gail was told she'd need to have major surgery, she decided she'd tell her friends about it. Sometimes she went to coffee mornings but wasn't very close to everyone there so only told one person in confidence from that group, wanting to limit who knew about her surgery. Gail had been warned there might be a long wait for her surgery and didn't want everyone asking her about it whenever they met as she was feeling very apprehensive.

By the time Gail had started to email friends that she saw infrequently, she added to someone, 'I'm only telling close friends so please could you keep this to yourself.' Later in bed, Gail realized what she'd written. If she only told close friends about her surgery, she could therefore count everyone she'd already told as a close friend. The number of close friends Gail found herself to have was amazing. She had 12.

It was clear that Gail wasn't in urgent need of new friends so instead she decided to put effort into increasing the level of intimacy she had with a couple of friends that lived close by to help moderate her loneliness.

Personality and long-term loneliness

For some people, loneliness is an old but unwanted companion. It goes with them wherever they are and can stay with them even when they are with other people. If you feel lonely much of the time, consider whether your personality perpetuates your loneliness (see suggestions below – also see Chapter 3). In facing up to weaknesses in this area you are empowering yourself to make a difference to your life – permanently. Identifying personality types that are unhelpful in forming relationships is the first step in changing the way you relate to others and by learning people skills (see Chapters 4, 5 and 6) you will be able to relate more positively to other people in the future which will secure you a good chance of forming lasting friendships.

It is also useful to see if you can spot similar personalities in other people as it will help you to understand why you don't like them, or why they behave the way they do. By becoming more aware of how other people behave, you are increasing your own self-awareness.

Unhelpful personality types

You will probably recognize some of these less endearing types – they are role models to avoid!

Being arrogant is a superior stance in which people may assume they are better than other people – not behaviour that others warm to! To make friends, such people would need to equalize the balance of differences and find a base of commonality – such as both enjoying football.

Being a know-all is another superior stance whereby someone may always be putting others down and assuming superior knowledge.

Being irritating can be frustrating for others. Irritating habits

16

include continually interrupting and not letting the other person have an opportunity to speak, which can be due to social nervousness; or continually reverting to the same topic once the subject has been thoroughly aired and the other person has shown a need to move on. Being overapologetic is also irritating.

Being insensitive can hurt other people's feelings. We've probably all been on the receiving end of the outspoken type, who says exactly what is on his or her mind without regard to who is listening. For example, someone who's just lost her job may feel resentful and hurt to receive an insensitive reply such as: 'You'll get over it' or 'Oh, you'll find another.' Such confidences are made in search of sympathy and understanding, not a flippant comment that dismisses the feelings of rejection and anxiety the person is experiencing. Choosing to change jobs at a convenient time is not the same as suddenly finding yourself with no job and the prospect of unemployment, or employment in a less desirable establishment.

When people feel hurt by something someone has said, emotional withdrawal is the most likely reaction; they will not seek that person's company again. Insensitive people can quickly get a reputation for being unkind and nasty, though it may more often be a question of lack of tact. Either way, it is best at times to keep those lips firmly closed and think rather than say.

If you suspect you are sometimes guilty of tactlessness, before you meet up with people it can be worth highlighting in your mind things that you mustn't say, and to consider safe topics of conversation or compliments (see Chapter 6).

Being unassertive whether through passivity or aggression may lessen others' respect, and the unassertive person will therefore be less sought out in social interactions.

Aggressive people offend other people, although in a gang this may sometimes be seen as a positive attribute among group members, such as at certain types of business meetings. Examples of aggression are being arrogant, quick-tempered (see 'Anger' in Chapter 3), sarcastic, patronizing, superior, distant, hostile and a know-all.

Passive people are too timid: being shy (see Chapter 3) and unable to take the initiative in conversations or to risk disagreeing with someone for fear of not being liked afterwards.

Assertive people have been found to be the most popular. They are confident about themselves, or they appear to be, which makes others feel relaxed in their company. They also show respect for other people and command respect by not allowing others to take advantage of them. (Various aspects of assertiveness skills are covered in Chapters 6 and 7.)

Being socially indolent. One of the causes of loneliness has been found to be that people are poor in adopting the roles necessary in social interactions, such as being a good host by introducing guests to each other or being a good neighbour by offering to help out in a crisis or asking after your neighbour's health when you see him.

But one study showed (Vitkus and Horowitz 1987) that lonely people were just as good at adopting social roles given to them by an experimenter as were non-lonely people, so they knew what to do but in real life did not carry it through.

So it may be that you are lonely because you do not value the hoops you have to jump through in, for example, making small talk on being introduced to someone new, or because you are not motivated to make the required effort in social situations, believing that it is not worthwhile. Here, a change in attitude will help dispel your loneliness.

3

Emotional blocks that hamper the development of relationships

People often build barriers between themselves and other people that prevent new relationships from forming, and stop existing ones developing to intimacy. These barriers can be lowered over time and may disappear altogether if you are determined to change the way you behave towards, and think about, other people.

Shyness

Being shy is a mixture of social anxiety, inhibition, reticence and social incompetence.

Being socially anxious is fearing you cannot live up to your expectations of how you should project yourself in company. This leads you to fear social situations and want to avoid them. Anxiety can make your social performance well under par as it interferes with how you behave with other people and react to them.

Knowing that your social performance was poor will give you the message that you are no good at social interactions and this will confirm any previous negative views you have about yourself, making the next social situation more anxiety-provoking (extreme social anxiety can lead to social phobia – see Chapter 8) and therefore less likely to be successful. You are then likely to be in a position of self-fulfilled prophecy – you always thought you were no good and now you know it. You will probably believe this even though the grounding for this logic is based on initial anxiety that affected your social performance rather than your inability to make friends and have fun.

Research has shown (Solano and Koester 1989) that anxiety in social situations may have more impact on loneliness than any other factor such as social skills deficits.

Being inhibited means that you find it hard to behave normally in front of others as you cannot remain relaxed. However, this may just be with people you don't know well or where you feel out of your depth. For example, if you have to accompany your partner to a work function you might feel everyone there is much better educated than you and that you are not good enough.

People that are shy from anxiety and inhibition alone – that is, do not have a social skills deficit – have no problem communicating when relaxed and in the company of others that are well known to them. If this is the case with you, try to deliberately relax when in new company and concentrate on how interesting the other people are. If you are nervous with some people remember that they are just people. Reduce them to a more comfortable size in your mind by remembering that they have bodily functions and needs like the rest of us.

Being reticent involves reluctance to communicate with other people, or finding it hard to disclose at any level. This may be a combination of not wanting to, and not knowing how to, share experiences and thoughts, and steering clear of social contact to avoid the anxiety you may feel at having to communicate.

If you are reticent you are likely to be regarded by other people as hostile and negative rather than being shy or nervous – so people won't be encouraged to make friends with you. They will think you are deliberately holding back any intimacy because you don't want to be friendly with them and they will think that you are not interested in the conversation, or them.

To compound this, shy and reticent people get used to not sharing intimacies and being open with others, such as easily admitting to similar experiences the other person has described, and through their habitual social failures learn to expect nothing more than disinterest from others. Consequently their body language becomes closed to future encounters, keeping people away. Practise letting people into your world, bit by bit (see 'Disclosure' in Chapter 5).

Being socially incompetent is having social skills deficits. This means that you do not respond positively to people in social interactions and they find you off-putting because of your manner, your behaviour or by what you say – and don't say. If you are shy because you have poor social skills, Chapters 5, 6 and 7 will help.

Negativity

Being negative about yourself can stifle spontaneity and give you a false perception of the world around you, the people in it and where you stand in the social hierarchy. In time you will fulfil your low expectations of success merely through displaying behaviour stemming from believing these negative thoughts.

Write down negative thoughts you have relating to your ability to socialize and other people wanting to get to know you. Some examples are:

- 'Why would anyone want to know me?'
- 'I have nothing interesting to say.'
- 'I'm boring.'
- 'There's no point in trying to make new friends – I always lose them.'
- 'People don't understand me.'
- 'I can't possibly invite anyone home. I'm too ashamed of the conditions in which I live.'

For each negative thought, write down alternative and more helpful thoughts that will aid your route to social success. I have made suggestions below but please don't read them until you have had an opportunity to try to work something out yourself.

Alternative positive statements could be:

- 'If they haven't met me before, why wouldn't they want to know me? Many people enjoy meeting new people.'
- 'I don't have to have anything interesting to say. But as I know all about myself and don't know about these other people, I can find out about them instead. And people do like to talk about themselves.'
- 'I'm not boring to someone who's never met me. If I see myself as someone who is interesting my conversation will become more interesting too. Most ordinary people seem to be boring on the surface, but when I take the trouble to get to know them I often find they have fascinating lives.'
- 'I shouldn't lose any opportunity to meet new people and talk to them. They might never become my friend, but if I don't make

21

use of my opportunities I may miss meeting the best friend I could ever have.'

- 'People will understand me if I let them close enough to me. It is only when I shut them out of my thoughts and feelings that they don't see deeper into me.'
- 'Just because I live in a poor area in a run-down estate doesn't mean that I don't deserve to have friends. I can't change where I live. True friends will accept me as I am and not judge me.'

Being negative about other people prevents you from offering and receiving friendship. Try to be open to everyone and suspend judgement. If you have definite views on whom you can and cannot befriend, accept that being so constricted has not worked for you, and widen your horizons. Part of the beauty of friendship is that it can be diverse. There are a multitude of things that can draw people together, and dissimilar friendships can have different strengths and greatly enrich our lives.

Having negative expectations about a social event, such as a party, will make you behave in a constrained and unenthusiastic way, which will dampen other people's lively spirits. You might also have unhelpful rules about parties such as feeling a failure, or considering the party to be a failure, if a certain number of people don't speak to you. You don't need to be the focus of a party to be a success – just to have met one or two people with whom you have had mutually pleasant conversations.

Fearing negative judgement from others is a form of social anxiety (see above and Chapter 8). You may spend much time critically evaluating how you feel a meeting or conversation with someone went, worrying that you gave a bad impression or came across as someone entirely different from how you normally are, making it hard to face these people again.

Consider how you regard other people who make social mistakes. Are you scathing of them? Do you always remember that error or do you go home and forget about it? It is likely that you judge your own behaviour more harshly than you would judge someone else's. So it is sensible to suppose that when you make a social mistake, other people probably won't think much about it.

If you think what you have done or said is fairly major, you can quickly apologize. As long as you recognize the mistakes you make, and try to avoid repeating them, there is no reason why you should avoid socializing and miss out on the chances of meeting someone new or deepening an established relationship.

Learn to make your social interactions rewarding so that you increase the likelihood of someone else looking forward to your presence and enjoying your company (see Chapter 5 and 'Giving positive feedback' in Chapter 6), which will help you relax and enjoy theirs too.

Anger

Angry people tend to have less intimate relationships than easy-going or placid people as they can lack the skills to calm things down, to see the other person's viewpoint and to allow for the possibilities of compromise.

If you are angry much of the time it can adversely affect your health: for example, a perpetually raised heart rate from suppressed anger is bad for you. Signs of repressed anger include being critical, controlling, cynical, aggressive, hostile and caustic. Eventually something will give: perhaps your health may break down alto-gether, or you will lash out with uncontrollable anger when the pressure has built up too much.

If you have a high background level of anger, you are less likely to cope reasonably with additional anger-inducing events, which makes you liable to vastly overreact to a situation. Showing others that you have uncontrollable anger makes you look ridiculous and makes others want to avoid you in fear of an uncontrolled eruption should they inadvertently upset you.

Anger builds walls between you and others because you can't talk to them rationally to understand why they have behaved in certain ways, or to explain why you have become so upset. Losing your temper does not explain to people why you feel how you do or exactly what it is that you don't like, so it doesn't solve the cause of the problem. It is also harder to make reparations following a big conflict so you risk losing friends and the respect people had for you.

Anger can be a positive emotion when handled appropriately for a just cause, but when handled badly it can be very destructive. Uncontrolled angry behaviour rarely achieves anything positive or solves the original problem: and you may have to live with the consequences of your actions for a long time to come, or feel extremely embarrassed by, for example, having to humbly ask for the job back from which you'd resigned in temper the day before. If you have a problem in controlling your anger you will need to seek professional help through your doctor.

Loneliness

Being lonely can itself cause further loneliness. When you feel lonely, you can feel low about yourself and start to think that there is no point in trying to meet new people because no one would be interested in you anyway.

In addition, the lonely get used to not talking to others and find it hard to suddenly switch into a sociable mood when faced with someone to talk to. The less you talk to people the more dull you think you are, because without regular social contact you deny yourself positive feedback (see Chapter 6) from other people. There will be no one to smile at you to show she likes you or to show interest in what you say. Eventually you may believe that you have nothing at all to say that would interest anyone else, believing that you need to immediately sparkle and amuse others to be seen as a social success: small talk (see 'Making conversation' in Chapter 5) may be totally beyond you as you see it as an irrelevance.

If you are not getting out of your home and doing things with other people you may also feel that you have nothing to say because you don't do anything with your life. Other people are not interested in hearing about your solitary activities unless they do these themselves. For example, if you love reading and meet up with someone who belongs to a reading group you may find plenty to talk about. But with anyone who is not an avid book lover, hearing about the latest book you read will bore them or, at best, not keep them sufficiently interested to maintain a conversation along the lines of books.

Elderly people who spend most of their days on their own can lose the skill of talking to others and without daily mental stimulation can become confused. They may repeat things or they may believe they have told you something when they have not. They may have so many internal dialogues, or talk so often aloud to themselves, that they may believe that you were the one they told these things to.

Talking to confused elderly people is less rewarding than making easy exchanges with someone who does not repeat himself or confine himself to topics that revolve around the prices of foods and household goods in different shops, for example. But unless someone is prepared to make a regular effort with an elderly person who is not able to get out much, her faculties will diminish and may mark the beginning of a gradual downslide of her physical health as well as her mental health. Try to be aware of everyone around you and be inclusive, even if you have not found other people to be inclusive with you. Everyone needs to have someone to talk to: long-term loneliness causes depression (see Chapter 8).

Unhelpful coping mechanisms in the lonely

It is very hard to admit to someone you have no friends, or few friends. Even young school children when asked if they have friends may immediately say yes they have. Even if they haven't, they can lie without hesitation as they already feel it is something to be ashamed of, something that devalues you, if you do not have friends.

All of us have been in situations where we have had no friends. When we start school or change school, when we move to a new neighbourhood, start at college or university or start a new job we are usually starting friendships from scratch and temporarily at least, have no one to call our friend in that environment.

If having few or no friends is a regular occurrence, however, people adapt their thinking and their lives to cope with their loneliness. But often the way they do this is more damaging to them than helpful in the long-term.

People can persuade themselves that because they are shy they are made like that and it can't be helped: that they are destined to stay shy for the rest of their lives. If their parents are shy as well they may say it's in their genes and so nothing can be done. Or they may feel it is up to socially confident people to make the effort to get to know them, as they are incapable of making that first move. Or they may feel that they cannot bear any more social failure and so learn to accept that they are shy, and the loneliness they are experiencing.

Some people persuade themselves that they are fine as they are and it makes no difference to them that they have no friends and so excuse themselves from making an effort to do anything about it.

All of these views are unhelpful as they serve to perpetuate loneliness and to make you passive – you accept that this is your lot and so are not prepared to do anything about it. You are powerless to take control of your life and seek something better.

But it is not true that once you are shy you must remain so. Becoming sociable can be learnt – just as your shyness at some stage was probably learnt. I was intensely shy as a child and teenager. But I have always liked being with people and getting to know them. I enjoy conversation. I wanted to do something about my shyness – I read once in a novel that shyness was a form of selfishness since we don't make the effort to be polite and sociable with other people and we expect them to do all the work; also, it is selfish to keep ourselves apart from others without letting them in. I would say that it is also selfish to ourselves to be shy – we are denying ourselves the warm companionship and support that we deserve.

Over more than a decade I watched other people to see how they behaved. I learnt from the skilful and the unskilful, which highlighted my own mistakes as well as helping me to avoid new pitfalls. I also learnt that even the skilled were not skilled 100 per cent of the time, which gave me heart. It also told me that everyone makes social mistakes occasionally; it is no big deal.

As well as becoming passive about their loneliness, people can develop other coping mechanisms, which may be harmful in the long run. Solitary pastimes, for example, serve a valuable purpose in keeping people occupied and preventing moping and depression. It is good to be actively pursuing something that you enjoy. The problem is that people use these pastimes as an excuse to fill all their time with their chosen activity.

Some may have a penchant for bird watching, train spotting or solitary walking, cycling or swimming, for example. Others may have decided to take additional qualifications through an evening class or through the Open University, perhaps becoming a perpetual student. Some people become fascinated with computers and spend inordinate amounts of time on the Internet, or watch vast amounts of television. Others may be reading their way through a library of books or have begun a hobby that they can do at home such as model

26

making. Some people may develop habits that create additional problems such as drinking, eating or shopping in excess and gambling.

It may be that you have put your life on hold because of having someone to care for – this may be because a parent, for example, genuinely needs assistance. But it may also be an excuse for you to avoid socializing; justifying your situation by telling yourself that once you are no longer needed you can get on with your life. But there are many cases where middle-aged children look after their parents and then find, once their remaining parent has died, that they are old and alone themselves. True, people have to manage to exist under some very trying circumstances, but unless you use every effort and opportunity to make contact with other people when you are tied, for example, to the home, you will not have friends.

None of the activities mentioned solves the problem of loneliness. Such activities may help compensate for so much time alone, but doing them effectively helps the person evade social contact, inevitably leading to more loneliness. The ideal of course is a balance, with time to do things by yourself sometimes, and time to spend with other people at other times. You may find that some activities could be done with other people, such as walking or swimming or joining a reading group to discuss the books you read. By making an informed effort on how to overcome loneliness, you can break the cycle of becoming more and more lonely.

4

Friendship rules: dos and don'ts

Different roles involve certain expectations of behaviour. A parent, for example, has 'rules' for how to treat a child, such as providing food, warmth and comfort; being married entails rules that if broken will threaten the marriage, such as remaining faithful. It is the same with friendships.

Some people are lucky in that they instinctively pick up what is expected in being a good friend, but others are left floundering, wondering why another relationship has failed or is not progressing as they see others' friendships deepening. So it can be useful to have friendship rules clearly defined, to help you identify possible problem areas.

Friendship rules

These friendship rules may seem obvious to you and you may think that you have known them all along. However, having them brought to the conscious part of your brain rather than having them in the murk of many experiences will make you more aware of your behaviour with your friends.

Show liking. When you meet up with a friend you should look pleased to see him and smile broadly. Making frequent eye contact is also essential. Imagine the difference in how you would feel if you were greeted by someone looking to the side of you while having her eyes lowered and her lips not giving the shadow of a smile. It does not make you warm to that person.

Close friends can often show loving as well as liking. This involves kissing on arrival and departure, and plenty of touching. Teasing and joking between friends is also very rewarding and shows there is intimacy between you: it is hard to tease someone you don't know, so the inclusion of this aspect of friendship shows that you have reached a high level of intimacy and fondness.

Be non-judgemental, otherwise you are putting yourself forward as being better than your friend. It is hard or even impossible to

29

make friends from a position of superiority. People do not respond kindly to a superior attitude in others, especially if they feel that they are being silently or even openly criticized.

Always keep friends' confidences. The only exception to this rule is when you think your friend is in danger – either from himself or from someone else. Trust is such a vital ingredient of a relationship that once broken it is rarely regained and certainly not to the same level as before that trust was broken. Divulging a confidence is a kind of betrayal and if you can't keep your friends' secrets, why expect them to keep yours?

Don't be too curious. Everyone is entitled to privacy so persistently trying to find out more about your friend than she is prepared to divulge will damage your friendship. Be sensitive to when a barrier comes up, then you should let subjects go.

This does not mean that you should never ask your friend questions or show interest in her life. If you never ask about the things that are important to her, you will come across as disinterested and uncaring. It is all about finding the right balance and noting when her barriers come up. Pull back when this happens. It may be you can return to the subject later on in your friendship when you have learnt to trust each other more – or you may never progress further than where you are now. This may be because your friend is unwilling to trust you and get closer or because neither of you are intimate with the other. Whatever the reason, you must respect her wishes about what she wants kept from you.

Notice when there's something wrong. Very often someone is quieter or louder than normal when there is something troubling him. Knowing how he usually behaves helps you recognize uncharacteristic behaviour, which should not go unmentioned. It is no good thinking to yourself that there is something up with your friend. You must ask him outright if there is something wrong and check his expression and tone of voice when he gives his answer. If he assures you everything is fine but you are sure he is lying, gently probe further and say that you are worried about him because you still feel there is something wrong and you'd like to help, even if it's just by listening.

Be ready with support. If your friend is in trouble you must offer support wholeheartedly. She will be able to tell by the sound of your voice if you do not genuinely mean that you want to help. Support can be practical – for example, could you pick up the children from nursery and keep them with you while she attends an important appointment? Or support could be emotional, such as listening to your friend and comforting her.

Very often support needs to be ongoing and this can be time-consuming. But you must be prepared to do it for the sake of your relationship. Some of your own needs may have to be put aside at this time. However, you are usually repaid in kind when it comes to your turn of needing help, if your friend is a good friend to you.

Sometimes support will need to be given in your friend's absence. For example, if someone else criticizes a friend and he's not there to stand up for himself, you could do it for him. However, you can only deny the truth of what has been said if it is genuinely the case that the other person has done an injustice to your friend by saying a falsehood. If the comment was true but you felt it inappropriate for this person to have made a judgemental comment either to you or in front of everyone present, tell her so.

Let the other person in. To get to know you, and for you to get to know the other person, each of you has to confide in the other and let trust build naturally over a period of time. Trust is vital in a friendship and the more intimate you are, the higher the level of trust required (see 'Disclosure' in Chapter 5).

As well as telling each other about previous experiences, heartaches and life errors you need to share your present world too. If either of you have had good or bad news this must be shared; your feelings about things that have happened and about other people also need to be shared.

Reach out to the other person. If you are in trouble and your friend has not gleaned this, you must go to her and ask for help. This might be in asking for a favour or in asking for advice: showing that you respect your friend's judgement by coming to her when you need help makes her feel valued. It also encourages her to seek you out when she is in need.

So much in relationships is about reciprocity. If you make sure that you do all that you should to be a good friend, friends will usually learn to do the same back by example even if they haven't up to now.

Don't overstep your role. Once you get to know someone well, you might feel more and more that it is your duty to tell him what to do. However, this will only distance you. People need their independence as well as co-dependence on other people, especially friends. If you try to take away the independent part of your friend, he will pull back. Generally, nagging is not well tolerated.

Show gratitude and appreciation. If a friend has done you a big favour this should be recognized in some way. Depending on the size of the favour you may want to offer to do the same for her or to show your thanks with a bunch of flowers, a box of chocolates or by taking her out for a drink or meal. Even then, what was done for you must not be forgotten. Be ready to help her when she needs it.

Some friends show appreciation of each other by genuinely complimenting them (see Chapter 6). By showing that you are appreciative of your friend's appearance, kindness or of the meal she's cooked for you, you are openly valuing her. In turn, she will find things to compliment you on. These things make the friendship all the more rewarding.

Avoid embarrassing your friend in public. This isn't only referring to being regularly drunk so that your friend has to apologize to others for your actions! More subtly, it includes letting out secrets about your friend or about something he said, and being critical of him in front of other people.

Allow your friend to have other friends and enjoy activities with them that don't include you. A friend is not someone who should be inseparable from you, which could be claustrophobic even in stable romantic relationships. Everyone needs freedom to spend time with different friends and do different things with them.

Although you might want a very close 'best friend' as school children often have, in adult friendships it doesn't work the same way as at school. Friends, and friendships, do have a life of their own. This does not mean that the relationship is not special – it is just a more mature way of having multiple relationships at different levels. If you give your friend time away from you, she will value you all the more.

Don't be jealous of other relationships your friend might have. When people are jealous, they are often critical of the person of whom they are jealous. But being critical of a person your friend likes may result in turning your friend away from you: he could take your criticism as interference in his other relationships and distance himself from you rather than the other person.

If you regularly have to spend time with your friends' other friends and you don't like them, showing how you feel could leave you without your friend. You need to try to be tolerant of all of your friends' friends, as he should be of yours. This is particularly important in romantic relationships. Showing dislike of your friend's partner is potentially disastrous for your friendship.

Don't betray your friendship. You've probably realized that poaching your friend's partner isn't conducive to long-term friendship! However, more subtle matters, such as lying to your friend, or spreading gossip about your friend, whether true or false, also can lead to a permanent break-up of the friendship.

Things that interfere with making new friends

As well as knowing what to do right, you need to know what to avoid, to give yourself every chance of making that friendship work.

Having a mistaken concept of friendship. Some people do not understand what friendship involves and this can interfere with developing meaningful and lasting friendships. For example, if you have a childish view of friendships where you believe that a friend should do anything for you and be glad to do it, then there will be problems. Your friend has the same rights and expectations as you (see Chapter 7) – including the right to say no to an unreasonable demand. She will not be self-sacrificing all the time and take heed of your needs at the expense of hers every time; she will need to set priorities and sometimes you will be lower down on her list depending on what's going on in her life.

There must be mutual give and take in friendships, understanding of each other's needs and a concern for each other's welfare. Also, friends are loyal to each other and show commitment: they do not give up being friends because it is no longer convenient or because the other is going through a bad patch with which they cannot be bothered to help out.

Having unmatched expectations. You might be looking for a friend with whom to share every spare moment or with whom to share all your secrets. However, the other person may simply be looking for someone with whom to spend some leisure time in going out to the cinema or to play squash and does not need or want intimacy. Wanting different things from the relationship can make it fail unless each of you recognizes the need of the other and is willing to meet halfway – you play sport with the other person and she occasionally listens to your life story.

Some people want a loose, casual friendship and others want an intense intimate one. Be aware that if you are offering something the other person doesn't value you may be better off looking for friendship with someone else – or change your expectations and be glad of the companionship that is on offer.

Being unrewarding company. For people to enjoy being with you, they must get something out of the experience such as feeling valued, having someone show interest in them and looking pleased to see them, and having fun. If these things are missing, you are not likely to make a hit in your social interactions (see Chapter 5 for help).

Being unable to make physical contact. If you freeze up when someone just touches your arm, the person doing the touching will feel rejected. It is a compliment if someone likes you enough to touch you – this does not mean physical sexual invitations.

When people are comfortable with themselves and feel confident and happy, they can usually get much pleasure out of touching others and being touched back. Although you might feel it against your nature to touch, or you might think that you are justified in touching only people you know intimately, it is good to be aware of the pleasure it can bring.

Being unable to show finer emotions such as disappointment or grief. If you have not had caring and loving bestowed on you, you will find it very hard to bestow it on others and you might find it hard to work as a team: to cooperate with others – and listen to their needs and communicate your needs. If you try to open up little by little, it will get easier and you will reap the rewards of people understanding you better and therefore liking you better. (See 'Disclosure' in Chapter 5.)

Being unable to trust. When someone shuts you out because of a lack of trust, when you know this viewpoint is not justified, it hurts. So if you do it to others, you know that it hurts them too. Not trusting others means that you don't confide in them: so they don't confide in you, stopping the development of a warm and intimate relationship.

If someone has broken trust with you in the past, it does not necessarily mean that it will keep happening with other people. If you feel that it has, ask yourself whether you used the early painful experiences to monitor your new relationships. Did you change your approach? Did you go more slowly and check at each stage that your friendship was being valued? Did you become more discerning in your choice of friends?

Fearing getting hurt. Some people are afraid of making new friends or committing themselves to a friendship because they are afraid of getting hurt. Unfortunately this is a risk you have to take because everyone needs friends.

It is understandable that someone who has just suffered his partner's infidelity or a painful separation or divorce or even bereavement is wary of getting romantically involved with anyone again. But you still need intimate relationships to support you and get by, and taking well-considered social risks is part of life.

Fearing rejection. If you have been painfully rejected in the past, you may be anxious about it happening again. The more times you have felt rejected, the harder it will be for you to meet new people as you will think the outcome will be negative: that the other person won't want to talk to you or won't find you interesting. However, as long as you focus on the other person and show that you are interested in her, she will enjoy talking to you as people usually like to talk about themselves.

If you have frequently been rejected you need to change the way you behave towards other people. Use the advice given in this book to get a more positive response.

Having a poor self-image. You may feel that you are not worthy of others' interest because you are ugly or have an unattractive body. Negative self-thoughts and negative views on your appearance undermine your self-confidence and act as a barrier to getting to know others. You are so wrapped up in how bad you think you look that you cannot be natural when others are around.

Try to remind yourself of all your positive qualities. These are not dependent on your appearance or on what others have said about you in anger or jealousy or for revenge. You have a right to successful personal relationships, just like everyone else: don't block yourself from achieving this. Looking through fashion magazines, or style and colour books, can inspire you with new ideas to try to help increase your confidence about your appearance.

Having low confidence and self-esteem. If you lack confidence and self-esteem you probably fear rejection and even expect it. When you feel like this you do not behave towards others as though you expect to be treated better so you are rejected, confirming your low self-value.

Having low confidence and low self-esteem makes you easily discouraged. It is also hard for you to show interest in others and conversations are difficult as you don't make the required effort. By learning social skills (see Chapters 5, 6 and 7) you can gain the knowledge of what is required to be socially successful and putting it into practice will show you that you can turn your life around.

Having poor communication skills. There are communication problems when you take no notice of the other person's behaviour, to determine whether he looks interested or bored, or of what he has to say. It is important to try to perceive his needs in conversation – such as finding a topic that he will enjoy discussing with you. It is also bad form to take no interest in the other person: to fail to ask after his well-being, to never ask questions of him and to change the topic of conversation he has started as soon as you can.

Another area of possible failure is that of your body language: what your voice sounds like and the posture your body adopts. If you don't give the other person positive body language messages about liking him he will not warm to you. Chapter 5 advises on communication skills.

Hiding behind a social mask. When you wear a social mask you only let people know what you are prepared for them to know and you behave in ways to meet with their approval, being on your best behaviour. This is fine for initial contact but you will need to gradually lift this mask to develop meaningful relationships. You know that you cannot truly say that someone likes you unless she knows a bit more about you than the superficial you, and you 'let your hair down' with her.

Lacking honesty. A lack of honesty on your part will immediately tell another person that you do not sufficiently respect him enough to tell the truth. For example, if someone admits to finding the evening class you are both taking hard and you don't say that you have the same problem, when you do, you are being dishonest as well as socially uncivil. If you were to admit to feeling the same way, it shows the other person that you have something in common which helps bind you together, and makes the other person feel better knowing he is not alone.

A lack of honesty in an established relationship can prevent it developing further. For example, when a fairly close friend asks you if there's something wrong, and there is, and you say, 'No, I'm fine', it makes her feel hurt and shut out – you do not allow her to get to know you better or to help.

Lacking openness. A lack of openness is, for example, when you tell someone that yes, something is wrong but you don't want to talk about it. This does not mean that you should divulge close secrets to complete strangers but it does mean that if you want a close and intimate relationship you have to be prepared to give some information about yourself. In this case, it may help to have a general response prepared, for example, 'I'm having problems at work' or 'I have some family trouble'. This gives the other person enough information for the time being and protects your privacy until you decide how much more you want to share.

Another example of a lack of openness is when someone has upset you but you keep quiet about it and sulk. The other person will either think that you are moody or that you don't like him. It is not helpful to the relationship if you cover up problems as the other person will not realize what he has done wrong and so is not given the opportunity to make amends.

Lacking tact. A lack of tact can hurt people's feelings. If you are particularly pleased with a new scarf or tie that you've bought and you show it to a work colleague who shows she doesn't like it, you will no longer feel pleased with your purchase. Similarly, if you are blunt with someone over his new haircut, he might feel dreadfully embarrassed until it can be restored to its former state.

Try to provide a neutral comment that neither praises falsely nor condemns honestly so that the confidence the other person has in the new thing, be it hairstyle, clothing or property, is not utterly destroyed. For example, for a bad haircut you could say, 'It's so different I'll have to get used to seeing you with it like that' or, 'It's certainly striking' or, 'It was very brave of you to undergo such a radical change. I bet people won't recognize you.'

Being negative by discussing depressing things, including all your problems, early on in a relationship, or too much in an established relationship, can stop a friendship forming, or can make an old friendship fail. This can be an unconscious habit. Try to balance conversation 'downers' with positive topics and some fun – and remember to allow the other person to have his say too.

Having negative attitudes towards others also militates against friendship, such as believing in advance that others will not like you, or being negative about yourself and believing that you are hopeless with people, or that with your difficulties or problems no one will want to know you. With these attitudes, you may avoid, or restrict, social activities which is counter-productive when you want to make new friends and keep up with the old. (Also see 'Negativity' in Chapter 3.)

Having unhelpful attitudes towards friendships will prevent you from making friends with a wide variety of people. Examples include:

- 'I can only contemplate having a friendship with someone who is very similar to me in terms of education, background, social class, income, religion, culture and physical appearance.'
- 'I have very high expectations of a friend. Not many can come up to my standards.'
- 'I don't trust people so I don't want a close friendship.'
- 'I am all right as I am. I don't need anyone else.'
- 'I'm not willing to get close to someone else because I am worried I might get hurt.'
- 'I like to be in control all the time. I am not prepared to have a balanced relationship. If the other person doesn't like that, he or she needn't bother with me.'
- 'I like to get close to people very quickly. I'm impatient when it comes to small talk.'
- 'I'm not prepared to open up and let people get to know me.'

Keeping friends

If you value your friends, you have to work hard at keeping them. Like plants that are uncared for, friendships can wilt and wither. Regular tending keeps them strong and healthy. For example, remember previous conversations so you can ask about things that are important to your friends. Remember when it is your friends' birthdays and help them celebrate – put the dates in a diary, and you might also want to note any sad anniversaries, such as the death of a child or partner.

Show your friends that you are prepared to be there for them for the bad times as well as the good, for example, when they are feeling low or unwell. There will be times when you have to put extra time into the relationship, for example, by visiting them if they are in hospital. At such times, contact between you needs to increase: it can return to your normal pattern once your friends' troubles are over. Don't be afraid to show love and care. Be grateful for any help and sympathy you get when you are ill or are in trouble and tell your friends what their care means to you. Let them into your life so that you can share your highs and lows too: be willing to share your feelings, successes and failures.

5

Communication skills

How we communicate, through conversation, listening and body language, is vital. It is through communication that we market ourselves and show other people who we are and what we are like. They can then form judgements regarding whether we match their expectations of someone they'd like to get to know better. The chances of getting on with other people are extremely high if you are a skilled communicator, and it is easier to make friends.

Making conversation

When we first meet people, we use conversation to pass the time, sometimes in formal surroundings where convention demands we politely talk to other people. If that has gone well or we have further opportunities of passing time with the same person, we use conversation to get to know them better and perhaps become friends.

To begin to get to know someone from scratch or to know a casual acquaintance more deeply, we have to rely on small talk which provides the building blocks for longer and more intimate conversations. Small talk with strangers rarely involves divulging personal information and is a vital part of casual chatting to simply to pass the time, or to practise your conversation skills, and involves neutral, bland comments on topics that are accessible, non-personal and non-contentious.

When talking to a complete stranger you have no knowledge on which to base your opening chat, unlike at a work function when you are introduced to someone from another department, when you can plunge into talking about what the other person's work involves and with whom he works. However, if you start to chat with a stranger in an environment where you have something in common, such as both waiting for the bus, it becomes easier and you can focus not on yourself but on the commonality of your situation.

You can talk about the weather ('Isn't it a lovely day?'), the long wait in the dentist's surgery ('How long has the last person been in

41

there?'), the crowded shops ('The queues are horrendous. If I didn't really want this, I'd give up'), the unexpected fire drill ('I'd just reached the checkout when the alarm went off'), why you need to get home fast ('I've got to collect my children from the minder – I'm already late'), how nicely the children are playing together ('Don't they get on well? I do like to see them playing happily') and so on.

What to say may be altered by the situation – in the doctor's surgery it is a complete no-no to ask what the other person is doing there! However, at the vet's it is not only acceptable to ask what's wrong with the other person's pet, it is actually welcomed, especially after admiring it and asking how old it is: you are showing concern for another's beloved family member. You are likely to be asked about your pet in turn which may well lead to more chat – and you can then leave without knowing anything personal about the other person or having divulged anything personal about yourself: ideal practice at making small talk.

If you find small talk with a complete stranger difficult, set yourself a task to talk to someone new every day. This might be a customer in a shop, the person who works at the checkout, someone you regularly see at your station or bus stop or the ticket collector, someone you recognize at work but have never spoken to before, or someone who lives near you. Most people enjoy exchanging the odd remark with someone else as it helps to pass the time in a pleasant way.

If, as a woman, you have been taught not to talk to strange men you might only want to make small talk with other women. But a few seconds' chat with a man in a supermarket, for example, with other people milling around is not something to be afraid of.

Disclosure

To get beyond small talk suitable for a stranger or for people you know only vaguely, you need to learn how to disclose. It is through disclosure that you determine whether there is substance to your developing relationship – something to identify common interests, experiences, feelings, opinions and understandings.

Disclosure is giving personal information about yourself to someone else, which is something that many lonely people have difficulty doing. Disclosures are most easily categorized as either high, medium or low risk for the purposes of this book, although in practice you may have a continuum of categories, or several levels like layers in an onion.

Low risk disclosure is giving general information that is already widely known, or which you would be happy to have widely known, among your acquaintances, such as your name and profession. It is information that you wouldn't mind giving to someone new after the initial very insignificant small talk. Examples include:

- personal tastes regarding things like friends, hobbies, music, food, clothes and films;
- pets you have;
- family members;
- what you do or don't do in terms of employment and what you do or don't like about it;
- how you find your journey to work or place of study.

Low risk disclosure is suitable for meeting people at parties or work functions or when on early dates (see Chapter 10).

Medium risk disclosure is giving information that is neither highly confidential nor involves small talk. It can include:

- your level of success;
- your general level of income or lack of it (you can comment on the expense of things);
- the things in life that are important to you;
- what you agree or disagree with in current world affairs;
- how you feel about events that have happened globally, nationally or in your area.

Medium risk disclosure is good for moving a relationship on to more individual, personal terms.

High risk disclosure is giving very personal information (such as details of your rows with your partner) or information that could damage your relationship (if, for example, the other person was shocked by something you did). It is information that should usually only be given to people in a well-established relationship with you such as a family member or a very close friend, or on a date where

43

you are both close to making some long-term commitment. Examples include:

- details of past sexual encounters/activities;
- sexual orientation;
- details of abuse you have experienced;
- mention of a pregnancy termination you have had;
- mention of infidelity.

Sometimes the risk depends on the circumstance and to whom you are talking. For example, talking about your upbringing is low risk information if there is nothing in your childhood that was damaging but high risk if you were, for example, abused.

Use of disclosure in making friends

Initial contact with a stranger needs to be superficial and non-threatening so that both of you can judge whether you want to know each other better. And, if you do, you need to be careful how you open up: how much of yourself you give away and what you selectively hold back. Getting to know someone requires a skilful progression of your confidences in line with what the other person divulges but over a period of time, which you will need to learn to judge.

Instead of waiting for the other person to lead the conversation and ask all the questions, show interest and ask questions back, which should all be in the low risk category unless the other person leads you deeper. Be prepared to volunteer information that is relevant without having to be asked for it. This allows for a more natural and fluent conversation that both parties will find more satisfying. For example, if the other person tells you about his job, tell him a little about yours and perhaps add something about your commuting problems, or your hopes for promotion.

Some friendships can blossom more rapidly than others, and this does not necessarily mean you have given too much away too soon. You respond to how you feel and if the other person is as positive as you, it seems pointless to put on the brakes to artificially suppress what seems to come so naturally. But you do need to be aware that sometimes too fast progress can result in your confidences not being kept as the friendship is not sufficiently established to honour what you have heard and told.

Disclosing feelings

You may think that if you reveal how you feel you are laying yourself open to ridicule thereby increasing your sense of vulnerability. Or, if male, you may feel that to be a 'man' you must not show any weaknesses at all. A man is more likely to have difficulty in expressing the softer emotions such as telling someone he loves her, or in saying something like, 'I feel very hurt by what you've done.' But being able to share how you feel with friends increases intimacy and allows others to understand why you behave in a certain way when you have problems, for example, so that they can offer support instead of judgemental comments.

If you are not used to sharing your feelings, try it a little at a time. Consider the response you get and that will tell you whether it is a good idea to disclose to that particular person again. But don't be overcritical of the other person: she might not have well-developed social skills and may not know how to handle what you have said in a positive way, such as by being sympathetic. Just because one person hasn't skilfully managed what you've said doesn't mean you shouldn't try again. If it still doesn't work perhaps you are not choosing the right moment or the right kind of person – or perhaps that person confided something deep to you and you didn't react appropriately.

It is through giving part of yourself to others that friendships grow, and understanding and bonding strengthen. Things you could talk about are:

- what you feel about something someone has just said;
- feelings of inadequacy, pride, hurt, anger, disappointment or happiness that you have;
- how you feel about being bereaved and your feelings about the deceased;
- feelings of isolation and loneliness you experience;
- the way you feel towards your parents and partner;
- how you feel about the way you were brought up;
- regrets you have had;
- your deep worries or fears;
- how you feel about yourself and your physical appearance.

Be aware of the environment you are in before disclosing. For example, if you were to tell a trusted friend that you were very nervous about your first day at your new job, he would think it was a fairly low key disclosure. But it would not be sensible to confide in someone you have just met at your new workplace that you are extremely nervous and don't know how you got the job in the first place – the person you confide in might work closely with your boss, or be friends with her.

Listening skills

Often how you listen to someone is more important than what you say, and if you listen well the other person will think you are great company even without you having said very much. Listening carefully in a genuinely interested way is a compliment to the speaker.

Positive listening skills can be learnt and by following a few rules you will easily be able to develop rapport with other people. How you respond to something you are told can make the difference between no longer having that friend and having made your friendship stronger.

Listening rules

There are some rules of listening which if broken could seriously damage, or even end, a relationship.

Bridge the gap between you and the other person. Don't emphasize differences between you, such as class, culture or social status, but find areas of commonality so that the other person can feel she is talking to someone who understands what it is like to be her. For example, if you have had an experience similar to the one the other person is describing, admitting to it shows that you recognize the other person's difficulties and acknowledge that she deserves being listened to.

Match your body language to what you say and hear. If you're hearing about something sad, look sad and serious and if you are listening to an amusing anecdote, you need to have a smile on your face.

Try not to be distracted. For example, don't fiddle with clothing, hair or a pen or look around the room or at your watch, as it comes across as rude and disrespectful.

46

Match your mood to the other person's. For example, if the other person has just had wonderful news, do your best to sound excited when you congratulate her even if you are actually preoccupied with your own worries; if she has had sad news look sad and serious as you listen. However, this doesn't extend to adding fuel to the fire when someone is angry and needs to calm down.

Don't be judgemental. If a friend, for example, confides he is having an affair, or ten years ago she was in rehabilitation for six months following alcohol addiction or has just had a pregnancy terminated, try to be understanding and sympathetic whatever your private feelings or you could lose the friendship. Try to understand what prompted these difficulties and decisions and how the person feels about what has happened.

Don't moralize. When someone confides in you he is looking for emotional support, not a lecture on how he should live his life. Telling him how he got it wrong will push him emotionally away and he will not come to you again with confidences.

Be supportive. Invite the person to tell you what is troubling her in detail and be prepared to discuss the situation at length. You could arrange to meet up again to see how she is doing or suggest you go to see her or catch up over the phone.

Be empathetic by imagining what it is like to be the other person in that situation. Imagine what life is like for him, what his hopes and struggles are and how he feels about things. You could say, 'I felt a bit like that when . . .' or, 'I was devastated too when I was made redundant.'

Be sympathetic by showing care and sadness that the other person is having a hard time. Say things like 'What a shame' or 'Poor you' to show compassion: you don't have to have any answers to the predicament.

Be careful about giving advice as it would probably be from your own perspective – it needs to work in the other person's situation. Discuss several options with the other person so that she can decide for herself what she thinks best suits her needs. You can start a discussion by making suggestions: 'Have you considered . . . ?' or 'Perhaps you could try . . . ?' or 'Have you thought of . . . ?'

Check that you understand what the other person is saying. Every so often, sum up what the other person has said to show that you understand what he is saying rather than what you think he is saying.

You could say, 'So, it all started to go wrong when your son left home?' If you have understood correctly, the other person will be gratified that you are listening attentively. If the gist isn't quite right this gives him the opportunity to put you straight.

Encourage the other person to open up by asking 'open' questions where giving a one-word answer is difficult. For example, instead of saying, 'Had a good day?' to which the other person can easily dismiss your interest and reply with 'yes', you could say, 'How was your day?' Instead of, 'Are you OK about that?' ask, 'How do you feel about that?' or 'What do you think about it?'

Occasionally repeat a key word that the other person has used. For example, if she says, 'That's when I realized he didn't love me' saying, 'Didn't love you?' will invite her to enlarge on that brief comment.

Don't be afraid to talk about feelings by asking the other person how he feels about something that's happened or whether he feels better about something that happened in the past. It will help you understand him and show him that you care. Many friendships and romantic relationships are forged by chance that has brought two people together in a moment of crisis. Being supportive when someone needs an emotional crutch will create warmth between you.

Give feedback by saying how you feel and what you think about what the other person has said. For example, if someone tells you that her brother has died, you must say how sorry you are to hear that. If she describes a view of a situation you don't agree with you could say gently, 'That's not how I would see it . . .'

Listen to cues you are given. When people talk they often drop in a phrase or two that hints of trouble or good news and if you don't pick up on these and invite the other person to enlarge on the comment you will be seen as insensitive and uncaring. For example, if someone says to you, 'Well, it's not as bad as last year' you could ignore the cue and say, 'Oh, good.' A good friend will say, 'Why? What happened last year?' The other person then knows that you are ready to listen and are interested to hear what he has to say.

Don't gossip. If you are told something in confidence you must not repeat it to anyone else, unless you think that person is at risk from another person or she might harm herself. Even the person who confided in you may later feel embarrassed about having done so and she might not want you to bring up the subject again with her. At your next meeting, ask how she is doing and if she gives only the briefest of responses, take the hint and drop the subject for the time being.

Know when to say no. Some information you may be given could be extremely disturbing and you may feel that you can't cope with it, either because it is so disturbing in itself or because it opens unpleasant doors of your own and you don't want those memories brought to the fore again.

For example, if someone tells you about being sexually abused as a child you may feel completely out of your depth. You don't have to listen to everything that is being said. You could say, 'Look, this sounds absolutely awful and I don't know how to help. I think you must ask for a referral to see a professional.' If you are able and willing, you could offer to accompany the person to her doctor for moral support.

These rules apply to whomever it is you are talking. The most liked and appreciated people behave towards everyone with the respect they deserve whether they are close friends or not. These skills should be practised at every opportunity – at home, at work, when out socializing or just chatting casually to people you meet briefly. The difference in the way people respond to you should encourage you to do more of the same.

Body language

The vast majority of information we communicate is given through what our body is doing rather than by what we say, so learning to consciously use it is vital in successful relationships.

When you meet someone it is essential to smile and look pleased to see him. Depending on how well you know him, your smile can be with your lips closed (known as a 'social smile') or with your lips open to reveal your teeth. Ideally, the smile should also reach your eyes if it is to come across as genuine.

When you say hello, the best body posture to convey welcome is to face the other person squarely, make eye contact and continue smiling while you speak so that the smile can be heard in your voice, giving it warmth.

Women tend to greet close friends with a hug and a kiss on the cheek, or a kiss on each cheek, depending on their culture, whereas men are more likely to greet other men with a handshake. Sometimes they grasp the forearm of another man with their free hand while they do it, depending on their culture. Men greeting close women friends tend to give a kiss on the cheek. If a physical greeting is not the norm for you, however, don't feel you suddenly have to start initiating one.

In conversation you need to show that you are interested in what the other person has to say by making frequent eye contact. Meeting eyes for a few seconds and then looking away briefly before engaging eye contact again is less intimidating than staring unremittingly.

If you are standing, interest in another person's words is shown by slightly tilting the upper part of your body towards the person; if seated, by bending forward with a straight back towards her. The feet of the listener are another cue as to how attentive he or she is – they should be pointing towards the speaker, as turned away feet can indicate a wish to leave.

We all make use of other non-verbal gestures to indicate attention. Having an open expression by smiling and making eye contact is one that invites the other person to talk to you and assures him that you are prepared to listen to what he has to say.

Nodding your head every so often shows that you are following the conversation, that you agree with what the other person has to say, and gives him encouragement to carry on. We may also use vocal noises of the 'Mm mm' and 'Uh uh' type.

Try to be as expressive as you can in mirroring supportive emotions you are feeling (or think you ought to be feeling) from what is said. For example, when being told something funny you tend to have a smile on your face, while looking serious or sympathetic for a sad subject. Watching what other people do when they listen to a conversation will show you that faces and bodies don't remain deadpan and immobile. A lack of this kind of social empathy is one of the distinguishing features of people with autistic tendencies.

Offensive body language includes looking over someone's shoulder or looking around the room while the other person is talking, which gives the impression that the listener would prefer to be talking to someone else or is desperately seeking a means of escape. Yawning is an obvious sign of boredom. If you can't suppress it, you can at least do it discreetly and apologize to the other person, giving a reason why you are sleepy: 'I'm sorry, I've been up all night with my son, who's ill.' Sometimes laughter can be difficult to gauge, especially if you are nervous or shy: many of us have had the awkward experience of guffawing when mistaking what the other person says for a joke, or, conversely, not laughing when a genuine joke is told.

Be aware of the other person's body language as well as attending to your own. Watch for signs of boredom or wanting to escape. If you think you are boring him, change the subject or invite him to talk by asking a question about him. Positive signals include increased eye contact, brief touching of the arm or shoulder, repeated smiling and nodding of the head.

When you need to leave it is sometimes difficult to extricate yourself from someone in full conversational flow, but warning the other person beforehand that you have a time restriction should make her sensitive to the fact that you will have to go soon and also gives you permission to keep consulting your watch without offending her.

However, some people need more than this, so you may need to give other hints. When it is almost time for you to go, pick up your bag or wallet if you have put them down. If not, play with something such as a wallet, bag or keys to indicate that you will soon need these outside of the venue. If you have a coat within reach now is the time to put it on. And if these things don't stop the flow then you will have to stand and interrupt saying, 'I am so sorry I have to go now.'

Occasionally this still does not evoke the required response and you have to start backing off and turning your body away so that you only half face the person. If this fails say, 'I'm sorry I must go, I'm going to be late.' Soften your leaving with a touch on the other person's arm as you say this and walk away.

6

Handling feedback

Feedback lets people know how they are doing, and is important because we need to know what we are doing right and what we are doing wrong, so as to adjust our behaviour accordingly.

Children need feedback to get a sense of the world and how it works. If they didn't get feedback, they would do exactly what they wanted without reference to anyone else and without realizing that there are other points of view and that other people have needs too. Throughout our lives the feedback we receive alters our course of action so that we steer more accurately between the lines of acceptability and approval, and avoid crossing over into unacceptability and disapproval.

Valuable as feedback is, however, there are times when it is inappropriate to give it. For example, if you have just listened to a long and boring speech, it is polite to clap at the end with everyone else. It is socially unacceptable to offend someone who has perhaps travelled a long distance and spent hours preparing a speech. A one-off event like this can, and should, be let go without direct feedback to the speaker. Any message that needs to be given will probably be received by the fact that he won't be asked to return next year to deliver the same, or a similar, speech and he may have gleaned from the unenthusiastic applause that his speech was not one of the best.

However, when you are meeting someone face to face for a length of time or regularly dealing with someone, you need to know how to adroitly give, and receive, feedback to gain respect and to maintain your relationships.

Feedback can be either positive or negative.

Positive feedback

Positive feedback is, for example, hearing something good about yourself or about the way you are doing something, such as compliments on your appearance, behaviour or an accomplishment.

Receiving positive feedback

There is an art to this, and some people find it hard to receive compliments graciously, especially if they are shy or self-conscious.

Don't reject the compliment. Many people feel awkward about receiving compliments and may upset the person by rejecting a well-meant bit of praise. My daughter did this beautifully when she was younger and more obstreperous. She was told, 'That's a pretty dress' and she replied, 'No it isn't!' Think of how you have rewarded people who have said something complimentary to you. Have you denied the truth of the compliment? 'I look nice? In this old thing?'

When you get verbal feedback, the best way of accepting it is with a simple thank you to the person giving it. For example, if your boss informs you that many people enjoyed, and were impressed by, your presentation, you can thank her for telling you – and you could add, 'It's good to know I got it right.'

If you don't agree with a compliment, again, just say, 'Thank you.' If you receive positive non-verbal feedback by someone smiling and nodding at you, smiling back in return is sufficient.

Ask for clarification to understand exactly what the other person is praising you for if they have given you unclear feedback, for example: 'What do you mean, I'm good at everything?' Then they can respond in a more meaningful way.

Tell the person what the compliment means to you. This is the most rewarding way to accept a compliment. For example, if you have big muscles that you've worked hard at developing and someone admires them, you could say, 'Thank you. I've started working out twice a week. I'm glad you've noticed the difference.'

If you are told, 'You carry yourself well. You've got great poise' and you have made a conscious effort to walk and stand well following your training in ballet as a child you could reply, 'Thanks. I did ballet when I was younger and I've tried not to forget my posture. Now I know I've succeeded.'

If you are surviving on a very low budget and someone says that you look smart, and asks how you manage it, you could give one of these responses: 'Thanks. I spend hours ferreting round charity shops, jumble sales and car boot sales, looking for bargains. It's amazing what you can pick up. I hate to look badly dressed' or, 'Thanks. I take off my good clothes as soon as I get home and put on old jogging outfits instead. I treat my best stuff as very precious. I'm glad to know it's worth the hassle.'

If you have just given a speech and someone says, 'You delivered that speech with great aplomb. Everyone was fascinated by what you had to say. I had no idea you could perform like that', you could reply, 'I must admit I did enjoy it – but I also spent a lot of time preparing for it. I'm glad you liked it. Thank you for telling me. It's made it worthwhile.'

Try practising meaningful responses to compliments you have been given in the past so that you are better able to respond positively and rewardingly the next time someone says something complimentary to you. By rewarding the person who gives you the compliment, he will be happy to repeat it but if he is unrewarded, he may not bother saying anything complimentary to you again.

Giving positive feedback

Positive feedback needs to be genuinely meant if the rewarding message is not to be lessened.

Complimenting by putting yourself down makes the other person feel uncomfortable. For example, if you say, 'I can't cook nearly as well as you' the other person may feel she has to reassure you about your cooking. If she's a good cook, she's a good cook in her own right – not just because her efforts are better than yours.

Complimenting with a neutral or bland comment such as 'nice', may come across as a lukewarm attempt that will not be valued by the other person and may even cause offence. People often use the word 'nice' when they don't think much of the meal or new haircut; it is too bland to be a rewarding compliment. Instead you could say, 'This is delicious' or 'That was amazing.'

Complimenting overenthusiastically can also get you into trouble. June raved about a meal she was given at a friend's house although she disliked it. Now she gets the same meal virtually every time she goes to this friend's house. She could have politely commended her friend, by saying the food was delicious just to fulfil the social expectation of praising what she was given to eat, and waited until she was served a different meal on another occasion. On liking this one better than the first she could have been much more enthusiastic with her praise – and her host would have got the message that this was clearly favoured above the other meal.

Complimenting out of politeness such as when you are given a gift is extremely awkward if you don't like what you've been given. Thank the other person and do your best to look pleased, no matter what it is – and if you're not sure what it is, say, 'This looks very interesting. What is it?' If you don't like it say something like, 'How unusual, I've never seen one of these before.' You are not actually lying but are saying something to satisfy the giver.

Complimenting with specific comments that are appropriate and genuinely meant is the most rewarding to the other person. Some examples are:

- 'I think it's wonderful you're able to talk to anyone. You always know exactly what to say, even with complete strangers.'
- 'Your place always looks beautifully clean, neat and tidy. Does it take you long to keep it like that?'
- 'You're always so relaxed. I admire you for keeping calm at all times.'
- 'Your handwriting is very neat and tidy. It looks really good.'

If you feel that some of your compliments are too bland, work out what you could have said to make the compliment even better. This will help you find the right words when you next need to compliment someone. Then take note of how the person responds and compare it to the response you would normally have got.

Negative feedback

Negative feedback takes different forms such as criticizing or complaining to someone. It may also be given in a non-verbal way, including frowning, yawning or shaking your head. This tells the other person she should stop her line of conversation because, perhaps, she is being untactful or insensitive, or she is divulging something that is meant to be confidential, or she is boring you. A shake of the head can also tell her that she has said something inaccurate: she can then invite you to put her right.

Occasionally negative non-verbal feedback involves a sharp kick under the table – my mother did this to me when I was a child. We were having lunch in a restaurant with her friends. I can't remember what I was doing wrong but I had not been taught about the meaning of this kind of assault and so I loudly said, 'Ow. You kicked me!' Effective non-verbal feedback is reliant on the receiver understanding the message.

Receiving negative feedback

When you receive negative non-verbal feedback it's best to respond immediately and change the way you are doing something, or stop it all together. Sometimes an apology is required, for example, if you let slip something you shouldn't have and your friend, who was the subject of that slip, is glaring at you.

When you are verbally criticized, your first instinct may be to become defensive and excuse the fault or deny there is a problem. However, this is not likely to appease the other person. You need to hear him out and take note of what he says, and then work out whether you need to apologize or to explain why the criticism is unjustified.

Ask for clarification. Before you respond to any criticism, you need to decide if it is fair, which might involve you asking for clarification so that you can properly address the negative feedback. Asking for clarification also gives other people the message that you want to put things right if you have done wrong and warns them not to say anything that they can't justify. This helps command respect from the people you deal with which will also increase your self-confidence. For example, if someone says that you're never satisfied you could ask, 'What do you mean? In which areas am I never satisfied? Give me some examples.'

Unclear non-verbal negative feedback can be hard to tackle unless you ask for clarification, often in quite a straightforward way. For example, if a work friend starts ignoring you, you might ask, 'I've noticed a change in the way you relate to me. Have I done something to upset you?'

If the criticism is fair, it is useful feedback on how you are doing and alerts you to something you need to change.

Matt

Matt's friend was in trouble but refused to tell Matt what the matter was because he couldn't trust him to keep confidences. Matt knew he was right as he'd let him down in the past. So he said, 'I'm sorry. I have had a bad track record and there's no reason why you should think this time is any different. But I'm worried about you. Is there someone else you can trust to confide in? I'm sure it would help.'

If the criticism is unfair, you need to defend yourself by directly addressing what was said. For example, if a friend says to you, 'You're always late' and you feel this is not true, say, 'I was late today and I'm sorry. But I know I was on time the last two times we met.' Now your friend should modify her criticism and apologize for having labelled you as always being late. Once you have agreed upon the fact that you are sometimes late, ask if this bothers her, which it clearly does, and promise to try to be on time in future.

Francine

Francine's partner asked why she always shouted at him over silly things. She replied, 'I don't always shout at you over silly things. I shouted at you just now because I've tried telling you about it nicely before and you hadn't taken any notice. I shouted to get you to understand how I feel about it and will go on feeling about it unless you stop what I asked you to.'

Regardless of whether the criticism is fair or unfair, you will need to stay calm at all times and only respond to the words spoken, not to how you feel about them, as that can let the situation get out of control. Likewise if the other person is not calm and calls you names, you need to put aside the name-calling and only respond to the actual criticism.

Giving negative feedback

Giving verbal negative feedback is often hard, especially when you don't want to hurt the other person's feelings. But giving no feedback at all when it is needed does not get the problem aired or resolved – you just let it fester inside you, without giving any outward indication that someone has wronged you. This can create problems for you in the long run – feelings and resentments that get bottled up cause stress and depression, and don't enhance your relationships. You may feel long-suffering and misunderstood – but whose fault is that if you have not explained to the other person that his behaviour is upsetting you?

If you leave an ongoing problem without comment it does not go away but usually worsens. Ignoring a one-off wrongdoing can make you feel bad about yourself because you have allowed someone to ill-treat you and get away with it, but you may prefer to ignore it because you can't face the conflict that might ensue. If the insult is repeated, however, it's probably best to take the plunge and talk about it.

Don't blurt out all your grievances at once. For example, you might want to say, 'I've had enough of always being the one to ask you out, suggest somewhere to go, ring you up, text you . . .' Instead, address only one point at a time: 'I don't like always being the one to ask you out. Why don't you ask me out for a change?'

Don't give your criticism by sulking or by ignoring the other person because he upset you. This does not tell him what he did wrong, so he can't explain his actions or put them right. If you feel the need to sulk you could say, 'What you have just done has really hurt me. I want to be left on my own for a while.'

Be straightforward but without personally attacking the person. For example, if your partner grudgingly goes to fetch the shopping from the car but smashes the bottle of wine against the door on closing it, you might well be tempted to say, 'Idiot! I may as well do everything myself.' However, this will only build resentment and will not sort out the problem. It also doesn't address how you feel about what happened. Instead you could say, 'I feel hurt that you don't take more care with the things I ask you to do.'

If you feel very uncomfortable about being with a particular friend because she never has anything positive to say about anyone, you could say, 'I don't feel comfortable listening to you criticize your friends. It makes me wonder what you say about me behind my back.'

Be specific. You need to be very clear about what it is you don't like.

Gerry

Gerry and her husband Ian both worked full-time. Gerry had to leave the house half an hour before Ian, but got home in the evening just after him. For weeks she'd washed up her breakfast dishes and left them on the drainer to dry while his were still left dirty on the table for her to wash when she got back from work.

Finally Gerry said something. 'I leave for work before you and get home after you. I manage to wash up the dishes I use before I go to work and I'd like you to do the same with yours. I am not happy about you leaving them for me for when I get home. You haven't even cleared the table. I find it selfish.' Ian apologized and said he hadn't realized it was a problem.

Giving criticism to prickly people is particularly hard as you know that whatever you say will not be well-received: your act of criticizing will be emotionally responded to rather than what you say. But just because the other person has a problem, it does not mean you should be long-suffering. Other people have to take responsibility for their actions and inactions, and if everyone protects them from learning some much-needed home truths, they will never learn that their behaviour, for example, is objectionable.

If you know that what you say will not be taken well you could start off with something like, 'I have waited two months to tell you this to see whether you would stop doing it of your own accord. The reason I waited is that I know from past experience that you do not take kindly to any form of criticism. I am not criticizing you as a person, but your behaviour. I am hurt that this keeps happening and for the sake of our friendship I am telling you now to give you the opportunity to make amends . . .' In this way you indicate that you have done your best to be fair and give the other person a chance. It is then up to the person how she or he responds.

7

Establishing clear boundaries

Sometimes in relationships you need to set clear boundaries in terms of other people's behaviour, what they can expect of you and how they should treat you. Although you might become intimate with someone, it does not mean that you forfeit the right to protect what is important to you. Occasionally you will need to remind people that you do have boundaries and that you intend to defend them. Protecting your reasonable boundaries in a way that will not offend other people is known as being assertive.

Assertive people have been found to be more respected and socially skilled, and less lonely than non-assertive people. They deal honestly, straightforwardly and respectfully with other people, treating them as equals. They never deliberately offend, are non-judgemental, always stick to the point and ignore comments that deflect them from their purpose.

Aggressive people, however, are arrogant, intolerant and domineering, and lack respect for other people feeling they are superior; they do not care what they do to achieve their goal as long as they get what they want. They are often rude and frequently offend other people by their behaviour and what they say.

Passive people are timid and apologetic, seeing themselves as inferior to other people. They dread, or try to avoid, social situations. They easily give way under pressure, agreeing to other people's unreasonable demands and rarely make their needs known, being submissive, tongue-tied and unsure of themselves and their rights.

Treading the middle ground of assertion is difficult, especially as you may be unfamiliar with sticking up for yourself – or recognizing that other people have needs as valid as your own. It is therefore useful to know what your personal rights are and that other people also have these rights.

Your personal rights

I have the right to state my needs. This means that you have every right to tell people what you need or want. For example, if your friend always chooses where to go at the weekend, say what you'd like to do for a change: 'I'd like us to go to that designer outlet as I desperately need something to wear for my brother's wedding. But I need to be back before six as I've promised Mum I'd take her to the theatre, so could we meet earlier than usual?'

I have the right to be respected and treated as an equal. This involves not letting people take advantage of you. For example, if someone needs an errand to be run at the office and a friend volunteers you yet again, you could say, 'I've done it the last five times. I think it's time someone else took their turn.'

I have the right to some time alone and for privacy. Everyone needs time and space to themselves. If you feel that yours have been eroded, you may need to claw some back. For example, if you never get a moment to yourself in the home because of the demands of your partner and young children, you could say, 'I'm going to have a long bath now. I'm locking the door and I don't want anyone to come and disturb me.' Check that your partner understands that he is responsible for your children's needs until you are ready to take over again.

I have the right to make my own decisions and take responsibility for them. If someone tries to interfere and tell you what to do, point out that you are capable of deciding things for yourself and are prepared to take any consequences that might result. If you get it wrong, that's your problem, not hers.

For example, if you apply for a job in a completely different industry and your friend says, 'I don't know why you're applying there. You'll never get it. You don't have the relevant experience', you could say, 'If I don't get it there's nothing to lose apart from the time I spent filling out the application form. And if I do get it, then they obviously think I do have something to offer. I'd prefer them to make the decision, not you.'

I have the right to say 'yes' and 'no' to others and have my decision accepted. To get people to take you seriously, you need to stick to what you decide and not let them change your mind, or they will do it all the more. (Saying no is looked at in more detail below.)

I have the right to change my mind. If the situation changes, or if you have thought more deeply about something and think your initial decision was wrong, you have every right to change your mind. For example, if you have promised to meet a friend after work but you feel unwell you can cancel the arrangement. Or you might have been asked out by someone but are having second thoughts.

I have the right to ask for clarification without being made to feel small because I don't understand or know the answer. Not being able to understand something someone says does not reflect badly on you – only if you don't get the person to explain so that you do understand. Perhaps the person did not do a good job of explaining in the first place, by using unnecessarily complicated words. You could say, 'I haven't heard of that word before. What is it again and what does it mean?' If the other person tries to make you feel small because of this lack of knowledge, it is the other person that has the problem – giving put-downs is aggressive. If he continues to use obscure words, he is also a poor communicator.

I have the right to ask for what I want and understand that others have the right to refuse me. If you want something, you have every right to ask for it – but you must respect the other person's right to say no.

I have the right to refuse responsibility for other people's problems. It may be that you have enough problems of your own to deal with or that someone is continually dumping troubles at your feet and you cannot face hearing about them any more.

For example, a friend might ask to come round because she's upset: she does this on a regular basis. You could say, 'I'm sorry but I can't see you tonight. I have some things of my own I need to sort out.' If she takes offence, and always takes from you rather than sharing the giving and taking, this may signal the end of an unfulfilling relationship. That's not your problem either; she has clearly overstepped your boundary.

I have the right to interact with others without changing my behaviour merely for their approval. You have the right to be the person you are without feeling the need to change to suit everyone else. Just acknowledging this can take the pressure off many situations where you might otherwise feel you had to act a part to win approval – meeting your new boss or future mother-in-law, for example.

I have the right to be successful. Although it is not a positive attribute to be boastful, it is also not positive behaviour to deliberately hide your success by being too modest or hiding your light under a bushel. Any success you have, when asked about, should be admitted to openly and matter-of-factly. For example, you could say, 'Yes, I did get a first in my degree.'

I have the right to change any part of myself. We adapt to life experiences and through them become more of who we are meant to be. For the changes to be positive, we should be improving ourselves in some way. For example, if your partner objects to the fact that you are no longer there to share all the evenings with her, you could say, 'I am not out partying without you. I am at evening classes because I want more for myself. I have the right to improve my job prospects and would be glad of your support.'

Asking for help

Many passive or timid people find it hard or impossible to ask for help. They feel it shows them up as being less capable than other people, or they feel ashamed of having to ask. But we all need help from time to time and most of us are willing to give it, so why not be also willing to receive it?

To have the best chance of getting the help you want, you need to be clear about what you want, and the reasons why. Ask in a straightforward way so that the other person is not trying to guess at the underlying reasons for your requests.

For example, you might want to ask for help at home. So be specific. Instead of just saying, 'Will you help me more in the home?' say, 'I am tired when I get home from work. I'd like you to help me with either cooking or getting the children ready for bed' or, 'I've got to finish my assignment today and need all the time I can give it. Would you take the children out for the day and buy them their tea?'

Sometimes help is offered in abundance and you may need to control it.

Marcia
Marcia's mother came every day to help after Adam was born, but when Marcia was better able to cope she wanted more time to herself and her baby. She said to her mother, 'I appreciate all the help you have given me. It's been wonderful. But now that Adam's sleeping through the night, I'd like to try it on my own for a while, to have the confidence to know I can cope. If it

doesn't work out you'll be the first person I call. Perhaps Adam and I can visit you for a change or meet in town?'

Asking for what you want

Asking for what you want can be very difficult, particularly if you are shy. You may fear that it sounds as if you are making demands, and you may feel it is not in your nature to be so forward. However, unless you let people know your needs you won't have them fulfilled as other people are not mind readers. Giving reasons for wanting what you ask for helps others to understand the importance of complying with your wishes.

To take a fundamental example, you might want to stop someone else from smoking in your house. As the person is lighting up, you could say, 'I'm very sorry but we don't smoke and we ask our guests not to' or, 'Would you mind not smoking? I have asthma.' Or even just, 'I'm sorry, this is a non-smoking zone.' If your brother-in-law swears all the time you could say, 'Please stop using "bad" language in front of my children – I worry they will use the same words and expressions.'

Sometimes not asking for something can get you into more trouble than if you had asked.

Hugh

Hugh had been invited to dinner at a friend's house. His mother was coming in the afternoon for tea but instead of ringing up his mother and telling her that he'd been invited out and asking if she could come either a little earlier or punctually so that he wouldn't be late for his host and still have time for a lengthy chat with her, he hoped for the best. But Hugh's mother arrived late. Still he didn't tell her about his dinner arrangement but kept consulting his watch. Ten minutes before he was due to leave he blurted out that he had to get ready as he was going out. His mother was offended and left immediately, feeling rejected.

Reward/penalty system

Sometimes, you need to give the other person a chance to consider the consequences if he doesn't meet your request. If the thing you want to ask is very important to you or your relationship, then you should use a reward/penalty system.

For example, if you have repeatedly lent money to a friend so that he could buy a drink, you could say, 'I'll give you the money (reward) but this will be the last time unless you repay me what I've lent you already (penalty).'

If your best friend told one of your confidences to someone else and you now find it hard to trust her you could say, 'I like you very much and enjoy your company (reward) but if you ever tell something that I tell you in confidence again I'll never trust you and it would threaten the future of our friendship (penalty).'

Saying no

You need to be able to say no when the issue is important to you. If you always capitulate and agree to things against your personal wishes, your self-esteem will suffer.

Identify the emotional beliefs that may be getting in your way. We tend to be brought up to avoid hurting other people's feelings, and to please people when we can. But, taken too far, these emotional beliefs turn into feelings of responsibility for the other person's happiness. Such beliefs can stand in the way of our own freedom to make decisions and to say no when we want to. So, try and identify them. For example, if you refuse to work overtime, do you fear losing your job? Once you have identified your beliefs, restate them: My boss may be disappointed but is unlikely to sack me out of hand.

Mean it when you say no. Very often people are forced into doing things or accepting situations because they do not like to say no, or don't say no in an assertive way, which then invites others to press them to change their minds. When you refuse something, you must not leave any doubt in the other person's mind that you do mean it. Use the word no if you anticipate difficulty in having your decision accepted. Using the person's name adds emphasis to your refusal.

Ensure your body language backs up your message. Are you making eye contact? Is your tone apologetic? Your manner needs to be quietly and confidently assertive as well as your words.

Practise. It may be easier to say no to some people than to others. So, practise saying no to people who you know won't mind, or where only trivial issues are concerned.

Ask for time to think. If you are not sure of what you want to say

66

or how you want to say it, try giving yourself time, by telling the other person that you will think about it. Then sort out what you feel and what your irrational beliefs and expectations are about your saying no.

Heidi

As a favour, Heidi offered to look after her neighbour Carol's children after school one evening because Carol was getting home from work late. Then Carol expected Heidi to do it every day. Heidi said, 'Carol, I don't mind helping out occasionally when you are in a fix, but I am not prepared to have your children every day. If you need regular help you must find someone else to look after the children.'

Tracy

Tracy was invited to a make-up party at a friend's house. But she knew that she would be expected to buy something despite her friend Amy's assurance to the contrary. Since Tracy was on a low income she needed every penny and could not afford the luxury of buying something she did not need. So she said, 'No, Amy, I'm not coming. It's very kind of you to invite me but I don't have any spare money and despite what you say I would feel awkward being the only one not to buy something.'

Derek

Derek was invited to dinner at a friend's house but was fed up with John and his wife trying to find him a partner. He wanted to be left in peace after his divorce. 'No, John, I'm not free to come on Saturday. I know you're trying to be nice but I don't want to meet any more single women. I'll happily go for a drink with you sometime to catch up on news.'

If anyone tries to persist in getting you to change your mind, say no firmly. You may need to repeat this, and perhaps add, 'I mean what I say.'

Saying no to sex. If sex does not feel right for you, then you should say no. For example, if you have recently started a new relationship and your partner is pressing you to have sex with him but you feel uncomfortable about this, it is important to refuse, rather than feel coerced. You could say, 'No. I don't feel comfortable about having sex yet' or, 'No. You're going too fast for me. I'd like us to know one another better before we have sex.'

It greatly lowers your self-esteem to have sex when you don't really want to or to get involved in something when you don't really want to. Going along with things because it is the easier path to follow damages your self-esteem. It also makes it harder to say no the next time you are asked. Or you might tell yourself that you've done it before, loads of times maybe, so you've lost the right to say no. But that is totally untrue. You have a right to change your mind at any time.

Conflict and negotiating

When two or more people want the same thing, such as the same holiday slot in a small company, there is bound to be conflict. Tension can also arise if, for example, two people want different things from a relationship – such as one person just wanting fun when the other wants to settle down.

Passive people avoid conflict and prefer to give in straightaway, but they will then lose out completely.

Aggressive people often thrive on conflict and stubbornly refuse to see the issue from anyone else's point of view. They may get their own way at the expense of taking advantage of someone else, or they may not achieve anything as there is a deadlock between them and the other person.

Assertive people seek to negotiate so that they, and the other person, get something out of the deal. They listen to what the other person has to say, then say their piece and calmly discuss whether they can come to a compromise acceptable to both of them. Then each side is seen to win.

For example, if your flatmate wants to get a cat or other furry pet but you're allergic to animal hair, you could ask, 'Could you buy a pet without fur? I'd be happy to look after it while you're away.' Or if you and your friend can't agree on where to go on the weekend ask, 'How about if I choose this week and you choose next week? Or the other way round?'

Throughout life you will need to compromise on numerous issues

– this is the way relationships work, especially in marriage and when dealing with teenagers! By becoming a good negotiator, you can protect yourself from being taken for granted. For example, if your partner always expects you to provide a cooked meal in the evening regardless of whether he is home to eat with you or two hours later, you might say you are not going to cook for him any more in the evening; he can get his own meal. Your partner might think this is unreasonable if you are cooking for yourself and demand that you carry on as you have been. You could arrange a fair compromise along the following lines: 'If you are home late I'll cook only for myself' or, 'We can look after ourselves when you are home late but on the other nights we should take it in turns to cook' or, 'I'll cook the nights you are home late, but you can cook when you are home on time.'

Handling angry people

When dealing with an angry person, your main task is to try to get him to calm down and listen to your point of view. This is not telling him he is wrong, just asking him to listen to what you have to say and then to take time to consider. Then ask if perhaps you can both discuss ways to find a compromise acceptable to both of you.

It will help if you behave in a calm manner yourself: getting heated will only make matters worse. Don't raise your voice. Speak slowly, acknowledge any unfairness in what the other person is complaining about and the need to discuss how to improve things.

Don't start your sentences with 'You' as this can be seen as aggressive and accusing and will make the other person angrier. For example, it would be no good trying to calm someone down by saying, 'You're too fired up about this. You need to calm down.' Instead you could say, 'Shall we talk about this calmly and see what ideas we can come up with?'

If someone says something with which you disagree, tell him. If he won't listen, you will either have to agree to disagree and leave it, or suggest discussing it another time, when he is not so angry. If you are afraid for your safety leave the situation and do not try to make amends: you need to get out.

Try to meet the other person halfway and show your willingness to do this by openly saying what you do agree with – angry people do need to feel that they are being taken seriously and treated fairly.

For example, if you were late in picking up your young child from school and your wife screams at you about things that could have happened had the school not kept your son inside and about the stress you'd caused your son, you could reply, 'Everything you've said is absolutely right. I am sorry. I forgot the time and then I had a phone call. I should have ignored it. And I'm sorry that my being late upset him. It won't happen again.'

If your boss is angry with you for not handing in a report on time, but you'd put it on her desk last Friday, all you need to say is, 'I put the report on your desk last Friday.'

Sometimes people are angry for no logical reason apart from what they are imagining. For example, if you are living with someone who is very controlling and is angry because you are half an hour late home, convinced that this fact alone means you are having an affair, you are not dealing with a rational person. People that are controlling like this may need professional help – if they won't accept help, you may need to get out of the relationship.

Put-downs

Put-downs are a form of aggression that deliberately undermine your confidence and cross your boundary of respect. They are hard for the unskilled to respond to, and some respond inappropriately by losing their temper. At times, they are difficult even for those who usually do know how to respond – we are more vulnerable to certain people, and during certain times.

If you suspect someone has used a put-down with you, challenge what was said to see if the other person can justify her snide comment – if you don't challenge the put-down, you give the other person permission to carry on doing more of the same to you and to others. For example, if someone says to you, 'I should have known you'd say something like that' ask what she means; don't let it go.

If you struggle over working out the change you will need at the post office and your friend says, 'Mental arithmetic is obviously not one of your talents', you could reply, 'I do prefer to use a calculator. Did you say that to make me feel small?'

Prejudicial put-downs

Since prejudices are not based on fact, question what the person says and correct any wrong assumptions – you need to be informed to put the person right. Some examples are given below:

> Your new neighbour says that all animals are dirty and shouldn't be allowed in the house. She is referring to your cat. You could say, 'My cat gives me much pleasure and, compared with most pets, is very clean.'

> You've just bought a new computer and have told your computer-illiterate friend. He replies, 'Using one of those will damage your eyes.' You could say, 'If you take regular breaks and exercise the eye muscles there's no reason why it should be worse than focusing on a book for hours. Computer screens have far less flicker now than they used to and you can shield the monitor to reduce glare.'

> You've been promoted and have to move to a different area because you'll be working in a different office and someone says, 'Oh, I don't know what you want to go there for. The town's a dump.' You could reply with, 'I didn't know you were familiar with X. When did you last go there? . . . Did you know they've completely rebuilt the town centre and its shopping centre has won an architectural award?'

A *racial put-down* is a special form of prejudice. Racism is believing your race or ethnic group is superior to others. You need to show the person who has been racist that his thinking is wrong. Assertively challenge anything that you don't agree with. Examples are given below:

> You are black and are with black friends. You all go to a pub and the barman refuses to serve you. You could say, 'I have never been in this pub before so I couldn't have offended you in any way. Please could you explain why you are refusing to serve me?'

> You say something someone doesn't like and he replies, 'Shut

71

your big Australian mouth.' You could say, 'I may have a big mouth but being Australian has nothing to do with it.'

You go to see a sad film with some non-British friends. At the end, they are all in tears, but you are dry-eyed. They say to you, 'That's so typical of the British. They're cold and emotionless.' You could say, 'Just because I haven't cried, doesn't mean all the British are emotionless. I don't tend to cry over films, but it doesn't mean that I don't feel any emotion.'

Stereotypical put-downs

Stereotyping is believing certain attributes and faults apply to certain groups of people, without exception. You need to point out the error in the person's viewpoint and inform her what the situation really is.

Sexist put-downs. Sexism is putting someone down because of his or her gender. Although most sexism is aimed against women, some is aimed against men. Sexism is a form of stereotyping: lumping all members of one sex together and giving them the same attributes. You need to challenge all stereotyped assumptions assertively.

Harriet

When Harriet's partner moved in with her she'd assumed he'd look after his own things, but he expected her to do all the things his mother used to do for him even though they both worked. Harriet said, 'When I invited you to move in with me it was as an equal, not my lord. If you want your clothes washed and ironed for you and a meal ready for you when you come in, I suggest you go back home to your mum. If you decide to stay, we need to talk about how to share out all the chores. I work too and I am not prepared to do more than half just because I'm a woman.'

Janice

When Janice cooked the first meal for herself and her partner, it turned out a disaster. He said, 'You've rather let your sex down, producing something looking like this and calling it food.' Janice replied, 'The meal is a disaster but I have not let my sex down. Being able to cook has nothing to do with what sex I am but practice and experience. I'm hurt you didn't at least appreciate the effort I made and I feel very angry about what you said. I'd like an apology.'

Bernard

When Bernard invited his girlfriend up to see his flat she remarked on a tapestry he had on the wall. Bernard told her he'd made it himself and she laughed. He said, 'Why did you laugh? Because you don't think the tapestry's any good or because I made it? It's very narrow-minded to think that men don't have skills that are traditionally associated with women.'

8

Underlying difficulties in making friends

Sometimes people are lonely and prevented from making friends because of underlying difficulties. Being stressed can make people just want to go home and be by themselves. Having problems in a relationship can isolate people from others if they don't want to tell them that their marriage, for example, is in difficulty. Or it may be that they avoid contact with others because of a family secret such as a son being a drug dealer or an addict, or a member of the family being imprisoned. Many people want to hide these problems because they feel shame about having them.

However, there is probably something in all our lives about which we feel ashamed and we should not be judged on that thing alone. We all need people and reaching out to form and keep relationships does us good.

Other difficulties in making friends that may require a referral from your doctor for professional help are depression and anxiety disorders.

Depression

Depression is more than feeling unhappy: it is a continued state of deep unhappiness that is experienced over a long period. Sometimes the depression is 'reactive' in that it follows a distressing life event such as bereavement or divorce. But sometimes there is no apparent reason for it. Common symptoms of depression include:

- being unable to concentrate or remember things;
- eating more or less than usual;
- feeling isolated and alone, feeling no one understands you;
- feeling sad and hopeless, despairing of anything ever changing;
- feeling tired and lethargic;
- feeling useless and worthless;
- having bursts of anger or impatience;
- increased anxiety;

- insomnia or excessive sleeping;
- lack of drive and motivation;
- lack of sex drive;
- losing interest in things you previously liked;
- not washing as often as you should and not taking care of yourself;
- overworking to dull your mind;
- suffering from multiple minor aliments;
- tearfulness;
- thinking about death and suicide.

Being depressed makes you withdraw from the world rather than embrace what it has to offer. As well as denying yourself the opportunity of having social interactions should you meet someone, you will perform socially in a disinterested way or in a way that shows you are unaware of the other person's needs in conversation.

Social pitfalls in the depressed

If you are depressed you are less likely to smile at anyone, make eye contact or bother with greetings. If you do stop to chat you might overinform.

For example, when greeting someone it is customary to ask how the other person is. However, this is very often a formality of politeness and does not mean that when you are asked it you should feel at liberty to launch into every minor ailment you have had since the last meeting. But if you are depressed you might divulge a long list of ailments (such as headaches, back aches, stomach aches, tiredness, etc.) because you are focused entirely on how bad you are feeling and how nothing is going right for you.

If you don't know the other person very well, it's best to gloss over minor problems and say, 'Fine. How are you?' If you do know the person well you could say, 'Not great, but I'm surviving.' If the other person genuinely wants to know more, this is the moment to ask and then you can give some more detail. But the way you phrased your answer also gives the other person permission to bypass that and say, 'Good.'

Once the greeting is over, you may realize you have failed to find out what news the other person has – you might have forgotten to ask or might have assumed that there is nothing going on in his life, as it is yours that has all the angst and heartache. However, this is often not true – I have found that when you take the trouble to listen, you find that most people have troubles and cares in their life.

It may be that you can't face being burdened by anyone else's problems in addition to your own, and so may avoid spending any time with that person once the greeting is over, making an excuse and hurrying off. However, then the other person will get the message that you are not interested in her or that you are too busy with your own life to bother with her.

Increased sensitivity is another hurdle for the depressed. A throw-away comment that you might not have thought twice about when you were well could assume great proportions now. You might feel very offended and hurt and think that this person was deliberately getting at you rather than making a joke that had gone wrong. It could ruin your friendship with him or prevent one developing, especially if you make a retort back.

Imagine a garden

To help with your feelings of desolation imagine your social contacts as your garden. As you think of the support they give you, plant them in your empty grassy plot to make your fantasy garden grow.

Plant trees to represent your family and partner, if you have one. The bigger the support these people give you, the bigger the girth and height of the trunk. These large trees give you shade in the summer and shelter in the winter, acting as a windbreak and a canopy to keep you dry. Place them in positions that appeal to you. You might, for example, want to plant your biggest tree in the centre of your garden, especially if your life revolves around that person.

You could plant evergreens to represent friends that are always with you and give you year-round support. You might want these to act as a border for your garden as they will define the limits of your garden and help to protect it from intruders, or you might prefer a fence to delineate the perimeter and place your evergreens in more interesting positions. Perhaps you will choose more exotic plants to represent some of your friends, especially if they are from differing cultures.

Plant perennials to represent friends that perhaps live far away but occasionally visit you or you go to see them. Assign colours and species to the plants these friends represent such as yellow daffodils or red tulips.

Acquaintances that give you pleasure such as neighbours, people you work with or meet through other people can be represented by brightly coloured annuals: plants that die after their season but with the planting of seeds and growing of seedlings can come again.

Make your garden as beautiful as possible. Landscape your garden to give it variety. A rockery, for example, can represent a major achievement in your life or a time that was bad and is now past. Let flowers and shrubs grow in it to commemorate the passing of the big thing. A pond invites other life to live in your garden and can represent the openness you'd like to feel for new relationships. Introduce new life by adding fish; you will soon have frogs too. Perhaps you fancy a stream running through your garden, and maybe a little bridge. Perhaps you'd like to separate the plants that reside on one side of the bridge from the other, especially if they represent very different parts of your life. A path will help you visit the plants for tending and care, and enable you to access and enjoy all aspects of your garden in all weathers.

Imagine your garden in all its glory and tend it often. If you neglect it, weeds will steal water and nutrients from the plants you planted and will grow up high around them to grab the sunlight, leaving your plants in the shade. If you do not remove these weeds, your own plants will become sickly and eventually die. The smaller plants will be affected first but the trees are the sturdiest of the lot and can withstand virtually everything. Your pond too may be so covered over in green that your fish die. Regularly check the status of your garden – if one plant dies, for example, because a friend has died or moved away for good and there is no further contact between you, seek to replace that plant with the plant of another friend.

Keep your garden pretty and healthy so that it is visited by the birds, bees and butterflies. If you provide the right conditions, your garden will thrive – as will your relationships. A flourishing garden helps keep you feeling positive and happier about life. When you feel down, visit your imaginary garden to remind yourself of all the good friends you have – perhaps sit under the shade of your main tree enjoying the warmth of the sun while listening to the whisper of its leaves. If you feel you don't have enough good friends, seek out more so that you can plant further shrubs until you feel your garden is complete.

Reach out to others

Allow close friends and family into your life. Let the people who care about you know how you are feeling so that they can give you support. Many people have no idea that a friend or relative is suffering and can feel hurt when they do find out, sad that they had not been trusted earlier. In life we all need a helping hand at some stage and most people are willing to do this for someone else – if they know their help is needed. It can also bring friends closer together.

Remember that depression is a serious illness that carries the real risk of suicide. If you think you might harm yourself, you must see your doctor to get appropriate help. Early treatment can help prevent the condition worsening and lessen the likelihood of having a long-term problem. If you feel your depression is interfering with your relationships, medication and therapy may help you respond more positively to people before the situation deteriorates making you even more depressed. Depression perpetuates loneliness as it prevents normal social interaction. Depressed people avoid other people and tend to become reclusive, so it is vital you do ask for professional help.

Anxiety disorders that prevent socializing

Many people would love to socialize and be friendly but are inhibited through fear that prevents them from achieving a social network to fulfil their needs. If you are affected by the difficulties mentioned in this section, asking for a referral from your doctor for therapy can help you attain the social life for yourself that you always hoped for. It is a big step to take but if your anxiety is interfering with your everyday life, you may need professional help.

Social phobia

Many people are anxious about social situations but when the anxiety is extreme enough for them to avoid the situation, or leads to a panic attack, they may have social phobia. With social phobia, people may be anxious about something embarrassing happening in front of others, such as fainting or being sick, or just making fools of themselves.

Although initially people's anxiety may focus only on their social performance when with other people, symptoms of anxiety that make them feel unwell can make them concerned about these too. Their fears then extend to worrying about other people guessing how they feel and noticing their anxiety symptoms, which leads to increased anxiety and consequently an increase in severity of their symptoms. Eventually this vicious cycle of increased anxiety gets out of control and they have a panic attack (see below).

Social phobias include fear of blushing, doing things socially with other people, eating in public, writing in public, speaking in public and using public toilets. Some people only experience social phobia late in their lives after, for example, a job promotion where they are expected to suddenly socialize with senior management, directors and important clients. They may also be expected to give speeches, presentations or go out to other organizations to train or talk to their employees. A job that they had previously felt comfortable in can suddenly take on monstrous proportions in creating fear.

Other people may have had anxiety about socializing from their teens, or even earlier, and it can grow as they get older because, as their anxiety mounts, they avoid more and more social situations. Eventually they can become a recluse. In extreme cases they may even have agoraphobia (see below) as there can be an overlap in fears about public humiliation.

If you are social phobic you are aware that your fears are not grounded in logic. The only way to improve your life is by increasing your social contact rather than decreasing it or avoiding it altogether. However, if you are prone to panic attacks this is an extremely difficult task to set yourself. Therapists ask their clients to write a list of their feared social situations in ascending order of difficulty in attending or participating.

For example, if you are afraid of writing in front of other people you might worry about them seeing your hand shaking or thinking your writing is inelegant or childish or you might worry about not being able to write in a straight line. You could practise writing in front of close family members, then close friends. You could then have cheques prepared so that you only have to sign them in front of the person watching rather than writing out the whole thing. Later you could try writing a cheque from scratch in front of people with whom you are increasingly ill at ease. When you are fairly comfortable with this, move on and push yourself to the next stage of writing notes to people or shopping lists (they can be wholly fictitious) while others are around, letting them get longer and longer.

While working on your desensitization programme, consider the thoughts you have that confirm your fears. Write these down and create more realistic thoughts that are grounded in logic. For example, for the thought, 'Everyone is watching me' you could think instead, 'People are not watching me more than anyone else and very often it is with disinterest – merely somewhere to focus their eyes while thinking of other things.'

Agoraphobia

Agoraphobia is a fear of being in places or situations from which you cannot easily escape. This might be because you can't physically escape, such as on a train or bus journey, or because it would be rude to do so, such as in the middle of a meal in a restaurant.

If you are afraid to leave the safety of your home, you are not socializing or meeting new people. If your anxieties include great concern about public humiliation you are made even more of a prisoner by your fears because you won't go to places where you are expected to remain a certain length of time, such as a party.

As with social phobia, you need to write down a list of fearsome activities in ascending order of difficulty and try to gradually work through them with the help of a friend or family member. People with agoraphobia often feel more secure if with someone they trust when leaving the home.

Panic attacks

A panic attack is a phobic response to a fear that is out of all proportion to the threat in reality. Although people with social phobia, for example, know that their fear is unreasonable they are unable to control it. As the experience of a panic attack is so awful they will therefore avoid social situations that panic them, fearing having another panic attack and being seen to be out of control.

Panic attacks involve numerous symptoms that include: sweating, palpitations, nausea, shaking, feeling faint, needing to urinate frequently and having diarrhoea. During a panic attack a person can feel so ill he may think he is dying or having a heart attack. Although it is extremely unpleasant and scary to have a panic attack, it does not physically harm you.

The way to overcome a phobia and the panic it induces is to expose yourself to the stressor in increasingly small amounts so that you can get used to one level of anxiety, reduce its effect and move on to the next level. Learning not to fight panic but to allow it to passively wash over you helps too.

Obsessive compulsive disorder

Obsessive compulsive disorder (OCD) is an anxiety disorder involving obsessive thoughts, such as worrying about contamination or that everything in the house is accurately lined up to your satisfaction, and compulsive acts such as repeated handwashing and checking that things are as they should be. It is very hard for someone with OCD to resist a compulsion and will result in extreme anxiety if the person is prevented from doing something he feels he must do.

Fears of contamination can interfere with you meeting other people. The thought of having to shake hands or even kiss while imagining the other person to be laden with harmful germs can lead to avoidance of all physical contact.

Having a compulsion to hoard can make it impossible to allow anyone home as there is barely room to move, or it is too embarrassing to allow anyone else to see the rubbish that has mounted up.

Being unable to leave your house because it takes all your time to keep it clean and in the order you need it to be to allay your anxieties also interferes with making friends.

If your compulsion interferes with your everyday life you need professional help as these things tend to get worse rather than better, and the sooner you get help the sooner you can start living again in the sociable world.

For all these anxiety disorders it is extremely helpful to be able to share your difficulties with sympathetic and trustworthy friends.

Suffering from these conditions also makes it more bearable if you have people to confide in; otherwise you can feel very isolated and alone which will not help motivate you to make the changes in your life that are necessary for recovery, or partial recovery.

However, there is a limit to what friends can be expected to put up with. If you are always demanding massive support, there may come a time when their patience is exhausted. Before this happens you should seek professional help so that the support they do give you is focused to aid you through the steps you need to take in therapy.

9

Loneliness in special situations

There are many situations that cause loneliness, or when it is harder to make or keep friends, and your ability to adapt to the situation and remain motivated is tested to a challenging limit. Try to accept that these situations are hard for anyone to cope with and be proud of any progress in making friends that you can achieve.

Going away to university for the first time is a very common cause of temporary, but acute, loneliness. Suddenly you are thrown into an unfamiliar world where you have no social support – it is a little like starting school for the first time except you don't usually go home at the end of the day. Also, you are expected to act more independently, making your own decisions and finding your own company and entertainment. You are completely responsible for yourself, possibly for the first time in your life.

Exacerbating your loneliness is the physical distance from existing friends and family and the emotional distance created by the fact that your friends are also doing new things or are doing similar things as before but without you, and that your new experiences may be hard to explain or describe to those left behind. Leaving home is a very vulnerable time and it is common to feel homesick and for you to increase your contact with parents and friends through writing, emailing and phoning.

You may make new friends quickly from your halls of residence, but these are initially very casual and may not last as they are friendships born out of desperation and fear. You may have latched on to whatever person or group of people that has accepted you, regardless of likes and dislikes or of personality.

In time you and they will meet other students through lectures and will establish some sort of rapport with them, making you feel sufficiently secure to drop some of the early acquaintances in favour of others. These newer friendships are more likely to last as they are based on areas of commonality rather than clutching at the first person who also needs a crutch.

Even then, however, your loneliness may not be completely

dispelled. New friendships cannot satisfy to the same level as old friends from home and at the same time those friendships left behind become shakier as they also move on to new friends and experiences.

Patience, understanding and acceptance of the fact that new friendships take time to nurture will help you cope. If loneliness continues, other strategies need to be put into place as suggested elsewhere in this book. When a large group of people are all away from home for the first time, they are all starting at the same point and are all keen to make new friends, so it is easier than when you are the only one.

Going to a new area to start a new job or move abroad for your work, where you may also have to battle with culture shock, a language barrier and racism, can be very daunting. It is more difficult to make friends when everyone else is secure in their own friendship groups and may not welcome someone they see as an interloper. However, if you make overtures of friendship towards other people, they will generally accept you joining them, for example, for a drink after work or for a night out.

There is a tendency for it to be easier for men to join an established friendship group or clique where all the members know and socialize with each other. Their groups tend to be looser and more flexible than women's cliques where they can often 'close ranks' and not accept anyone new.

Separation and divorce are painful causes of loneliness that have more heartache attached to them than just the loneliness itself, which may make the experience of feeling alone all the worse – there are so many memories that have been shared and so many everyday tasks.

Children, no matter how much you love them, prevent you from living life as you knew it before you had a family. Now you cannot go out as the whim takes you, you have to plan for it and perhaps even cancel dates because of a child being unwell or because you cannot get a babysitter.

However, since so many families have split there are now more people who are willing to take on someone else's family to form a new one. With determination, continued effort, and hopefully the support of your former partner, it can be possible to meet new people and forge a new life.

Bereavement. The death of a partner, friend or relation can make you feel acutely lonely, as can the loss of someone through moving or emigration. Although no one can ever replace them, over years it is possible to adjust to the loss and to find new relationships. When you lose someone special it is unlikely that you see anyone else in the same light, but that does not mean you should write off anyone new altogether. Try to be patient and open to possibilities.

A *lack of money* can prevent you from going out and meeting people, or from joining in with a group of friends that have a larger disposable income. It can also prevent you from travelling to a large town if you live in an isolated spot, which in itself can make you lonely because of the lack of people or the lack of people your age and age-appropriate things to do. If you can find someone else in a similar situation to you, you can enjoy each other's company without cost. Also, Internet chat rooms get you beyond your physical boundaries to meet people at low cost.

Being ill may prevent you from enjoying things others take for granted. And, if you are not feeling well, you are less likely to respond in a positive way to other people – you might feel irritable or grumpy or sorry for yourself. These are secondary barriers to the physical barrier of being too ill to leave your home to see people or to go out to work.

By recognizing how being ill is affecting your ability to maintain relationships, you can try to see people on 'good' days, or times of the day when you are at your best, to limit your pessimism and negative behaviour when with them. Try not to dwell on your own troubles but show interest in theirs. And, if you don't feel up to seeing people, you can keep in touch by letter, email or phone.

Having a traumatic experience that no one else has had can make you feel isolated by the fact that you have no one that remotely understands how you feel. You may also consider that the experience has altered you in some way, making it hard to relate to people on the same level that you used to, and that you now feel alien to yourself as well as others. If you feel like this, you should seek professional help through your doctor.

Being elderly can make you more reliant on people coming to you, and it is a sad fact that becoming older may involve the loss of your friends. My grandmother was the last of her group, being 98 when she died, and having survived her husband by 35 years.

To prevent some of old age loneliness, try to make new friends throughout your life in generations other than your own. (My own friendships currently vary from having friends 16 years younger than I to 40 years older.)

Working in certain jobs can be lonely. You might work nights and sleep in the day; or you may need to go to bed early every night so that you can get up early to work, for example, as a post deliverer. Or you may be doing a very solitary job such as farming which also ties you to the land at various times of the year, or to your animals that need daily care. Or you might be tied to the home with young children. Here there are, of course, others in the same position but you might not necessarily meet any of them until your child is old enough to attend nursery and you might always be socializing with children in tow.

Being homosexual or bisexual may invite negative attention from others as they display their prejudices. It is easy for others to shun you without taking the trouble to get to know you or find out what you are really like. Instead they judge you before you have a chance to make friends. This is probably why many non-heterosexuals gravitate towards big cities where people as a whole seem to be more open-minded and accepting of all differences to the majority. It is also easier to find others in the same position as you to befriend and form romantic attachments. (For help in dealing with some prejudices and stereotypes see Chapter 7.)

Being of a different social class to the majority around you is another example of prejudice that interferes with the formation of friendships. If you don't speak like other people or have the same level of education you immediately stand out as being different. However, the kind of people that this matters to may not be the kind that you would want to become friends with in any case. And whichever group you think you belong to, you could be losing out if you are too particular with whom you mix.

Being of a different race to the majority around you can also be very isolating which is why living in large towns or cities where there is a greater chance of finding other people with similar values, experiences and ways of living is often preferable to living in small towns and villages. Good friends can be found in any race so don't assume that everyone is racist about you – be open to new possibilities. (For help in dealing with racial prejudice, see Chapter 7.)

When friendships change

Friendships can change when something in your life, or the other person's life, alters. Some examples are given below.

Becoming unemployed through dismissal, redundancy or retirement loses you the status you had in your employment and the close link you may have had with the people you worked with. Although initially you might meet to keep up with the work gossip, in time employees will change and so can the bosses. With a change in management there can be big changes in the workplace and soon you may feel totally out of touch with friends you left behind.

Having an accident and not making a full recovery, or being in hospital for a prolonged time can cut you off from friends. If your accident has made you incapable of working or of doing the same job as you were doing before, you may feel that you no longer have worth which will affect how you respond to your friends.

Not being in the same job can put up barriers between your work colleagues and you – they may be embarrassed to visit you or to talk about aspects of their job that they would have previously shared with you, being too aware of what you have lost.

Having to learn how to live your life from a disabled perspective can isolate and frustrate you and you may no longer be able to share the activities you used to participate in with your friends – so you might have to work at making new friends who are happy to share in what you can do.

When a close friend marries you will find that, even from the time of engagement, your friendship thins. There is so much to prepare before a wedding and so much after that you can feel left out – by perhaps not having gone through marriage yourself and because your friend now has so little time for you.

It is only natural that a couple newly in love will want to spend all their spare time together so you will need to be patient and see if, once your friend has the wedding and any house moves out of the way, what the new ground rules are for meeting up. You might be more likely to meet on a work night instead of a weekend and almost certainly not a Friday or Saturday evening when you may be at your loneliest. Try to prepare for this happening as soon as you notice a reduction in frequency of meeting by increasing your involvement with other friends.

When a friend has a baby her time can be wholly taken up with caring for the new child and conversation may purely revolve around feeds, sleep and nappy changes. Being unable to share the experiences of this world can make you feel marginalized and the fact that your friend no longer seems interested in sharing your world can be a double blow. In time, things might improve but they are unlikely to be the same as before the birth, and very often people have more than one child to make their family complete so your interests may further diverge. However, if you were to take an active interest in the baby, you could do things together that tie in with family life and just take a different path with your relationship.

Losing a twin (or other multiple). The relationship between twins is a very special one. Unless twins have been encouraged from an early age to have independent lives, which may be harder if the twins are identical, they can rely on each other too much for emotional support and for a life companion. If one twin marries, for example, and the other doesn't, it can be very hard for both twins to live in a different house, and in some cases not share a room anymore. The spouse of the married twin can be annoyed that the unmarried twin is always there or always on the phone, interfering with their intimacy as a couple.

If one twin dies the loss can be enormous, particularly for identical twins. They have not only lost a sibling, they feel they have also lost a part of themselves. The loss is harder to bear if their entire lives revolved around their twin. The surviving twin may need specialist support from professionals used to dealing with twin and multiple birth bereavements. To protect against this possibility don't rely too much on your twin – develop other friendships too.

When you find out something about your friend that shocks or disturbs you, it can change your relationship forever and can make you question your inner self and your life values. For example, if you find out that your friend has committed a criminal act, you might question everything this person ever said to you, any advice you might have taken and remember all the times you shared together and feel sickened by it. You might question your own judgement – how could you have not known the true nature of this person?

It may be that you are not sufficiently shocked or outraged by what your friend did to end the relationship, but it may have soured it so that you feel compelled to offer continuing support in his time of need but pull back from intimacy. Over time, your friendship may die or it may recover depending on how your mind adapts to the facts of the situation. Often, after thinking about something over a period of time, the thing becomes less terrible and more understandable and so you may feel that there is still something worthwhile for you to hang on to. Much of it may depend on your own personal values and your own perspective.

10

Taking friendship further

It may be that you have an overwhelming desire for a long-term partner. You might have plenty of friends but lack that one important person who will make all the difference. This person may be an existing friend with whom you wish to take intimacy to its limits or someone new.

Although for ease of writing this chapter I have assumed heterosexual relationships, the same advice can be given to homosexual relationships.

Increasing intimacy

There are many ways to show that you want the relationship to progress to a romantic relationship. Increased frequency of meeting shows that you enjoy being in the other person's company, and laughing and smiling a great deal helps reinforce that. Prolonged eye contact, brief touches and the sharing of secrets can deepen your friendship and develop mutual dependence for emotional support and someone to do things with.

Look for similar behaviour on the other person's part to gauge if he feels the same way about you. Tell him that you enjoy his company as well as showing him, and tell him that you miss him when you are apart. If he feels the same way about you, this is an opportunity for him to let you know. If he doesn't, ask how he feels about you. However, if you are both too shy to show how you feel despite mutual attraction, the relationship may not get beyond friendship.

If he does feel the same way about you as you feel about him, you can then take the relationship into more intimate domains. If he doesn't feel the same way about you, be careful that you pull back and don't push him. He will feel uncomfortable with the friendship if he thinks you are coming on too strong or are hurt by his rejection – it could embarrass him. It is important not to lose your friendship. In time he might change his mind, but if it looks like he will never be romantically interested in you, you must look elsewhere.

Finding partners

If you do not have a particularly thriving social life, this may be something to address in general terms. Sometimes you need more specific help to increase the odds of meeting your ideal partner, by using the help of agencies or the Internet.

Introduction agencies can help to increase your social life generally by putting on events that allow you to meet many other single people. So you may make new friends even if you don't find your ideal partner. The social events could be parties, dinner parties, weekend breaks, walking, cycling or theatre trips and holidays.

They can also provide a speed dating service where you can meet many people – up to around 30 – in one evening. You have three minutes to chat to a person before being moved on to the next. This method of introduction can be useful since most people make up their minds whether they like someone in under a minute so it gives you a good overview of a large selection of people. You will be given a card on which to enter details after you meet each person to remind you which ones you liked and, at the end of the evening, you can submit your dating preferences. The other person is asked if she would be prepared to meet with you if she hasn't already included you in her list of preferences. If she agrees, you can have more time to tell whether you do like each other.

Some agencies are dedicated to matching you with a suitable partner. You will need to fill in a questionnaire outlining your tastes, hobbies and personality, and what you are seeking in the other person. There is a better likelihood of finding a match in a city since there will be so many more people out there who might fit your requirements. However, the pickier you are with how you view your ideal partner, the less likely it is that you will find him. Try to be realistic. For example, if you are in your late 30s, ruling out anyone who is divorced can reduce your chances considerably.

Some agencies offer particular specialities. For example, you may want to meet a highly professional person to match your own level of career or you may want to meet people of a certain culture or religion. These would be good if you are a minority seeking another minority. However, the number of people available to match you with would be relatively small, bearing in mind that you want to find someone of a suitable age, personality and with interests that complement your own. You have more chance of finding someone with a large and more general agency if you don't mind so much about the other person's background.

Some agencies match you by computer and you can request and pay for sets of matches over the Internet and communicate anonymously with these matches via the agency service. For example, Dateline does this. It offers two services – online and offline. The online is cheaper as their costs are much reduced if all the transactions are done over the Internet.

Look in your *Yellow Pages* telephone directory under 'Introduction Agencies' to find local and national agencies offering a variety of services.

Internet chat rooms. Some people prefer the complete anonymity of the Internet in making contact with new people via a pseudonym that gains them entry to a chat room.

Daniel

Daniel chose this method of meeting his new partner, Julie. Having been married and divorced, yet still shy, Daniel felt more at ease with approaching someone anonymously and without pressure. Over a very long period, they began talking on the phone. After many months more of calling each other they agreed to meet. As so much groundwork had been done up to then, they knew each other better than is usual in a friendship. Even so, it was still scary for both Daniel and Julie to meet in the flesh, photographs not necessarily doing justice to their true appearance. With that final hurdle over, they began dating properly and have now moved in together.

Lonely hearts. There are frequently columns in local newspapers that have free advertising for homosexual and heterosexual dating and also for finding new friends. If you want to respond to an advert that you have read, you usually have to ring a certain phone number and leave a message with your contact telephone number. The person who put in the advert then rings up a number to access the messages, and pays a premium rate for the privilege, which is how the newspaper profits from the service it is providing.

If you are nervous about dating, you could place an advert, or respond to someone else's, regarding friendship. Read the kinds of adverts that other people have put in to decide how to word your own. You need to think very carefully about what information you give and whether it is likely to attract the kind of person you would like to meet.

Casual encounters. It may be that you are out for the evening with friends and get chatting to someone to whom you are attracted, or happen to chat to someone on the bus you're on and want to take it further. Whenever you are out, be open to the possibility of meeting someone you'd very much like to get to know better. Going around with your head bowed and never raising your eyes from the floor to meet another person's eyes may get you exactly what you've been getting up to now – nothing! You do need to be a little bold to engage in conversation with someone else.

Under your nose. Sometimes when you are looking for something you find it was 'under your nose' all the time. The same can be true of romance. Take an interest in the people in your life and be open to possibilities. It may be that there is someone you quite like who is also attracted to you, but is too shy to make the first move.

I was very shy with people I didn't know well and so was a man I worked with. He started turning up in the prep room next to where I'd just been teaching after the last lesson on a Friday afternoon, and I kept offering to give him a lift home. Sometimes I'd go in with him for a drink and a chat. But it wasn't going anywhere.

Eventually I plucked up the courage to ask him out. I think I had to ask for the second date too. But he did manage to ask me to marry him. And, at the time of writing this book, 17 years later, we are still married.

Sometimes even the shy need to push themselves that little bit harder out of their comfort zone and take the plunge of making the first move. If you are worried about being rejected, make it a casual offer of going for a drink that any friend might make. If that goes well, you can make your intentions clear later.

Meeting partners

Social safety. Do not invite a complete stranger to your home or allow the person to pick you up from home. Meet somewhere anonymous and busy like a pub or café in a large town or city, and preferably in the daytime so that the date is less pressurized and more casual – you can leave at any time. There is an implication in an evening date that you will spend the entire evening with the other person – and exactly when the evening is meant to end is ambiguous.

Give your date a mobile phone number rather than a landline number, which can identify the region in which you live – they have the added advantage of being able to forewarn you about who is on the other end. Caller display services for landlines can be expensive.

Bear in mind that it may not always be safe to leave your drink unattended, especially if you feel dubious about the company you find yourself in. Men, as well as women, can be the targets of spiked drinks.

Be aware that some people may pose as single for the purpose of having affairs outside a stable relationship. Be alerted if someone has difficulties meeting up at a time when he would be expected to be with his family.

Women dating men. Dress in a feminine way but avoid very short skirts, very low tops and bright red colouring. You want to look alluring without being tarty, or the men you see may well get the wrong message and think you are looking for sex rather than romance. Go easy on the make-up too. Aim for a look that shows you've made an effort – but an understated effort, one that does not make obvious the time and trouble you have gone to.

Men dating women. Clothes should be smart and clean, and you should look well-groomed. Very casual clothes, cardigans that your mum bought you, and cartoon images on any part of your clothing are all probably best avoided, as are open shirts exposing a hairy chest and medallion, and brightly coloured shirts and ties.

Dating conversation

Once you have dealt with the small talk, such as how you reached the meeting place, you need to chat to find out about each other and find some areas of commonality such as your line of work, your family interests, your love of pets, places you have travelled to and would like to travel to, and how you spend your free time.

Try to ensure that the conversation is divided more or less equally between you. If you are shy it might be hard for you to contribute but, even if it takes a huge effort, saying something lets the other person get to know who you are. Shy people need more time than other people to relax and behave more naturally in a pressured situation like a date.

If the other person seems quiet, try to encourage him to speak by asking questions that require more than a yes/no answer (see 'Listening skills' in Chapter 5).

If the other person dominates the conversation, make allowances for first meeting nerves. Very often when people are nervous they gabble, and feel they must fill any silences, or not allow silences to occur in the first place. So although the other person may appear boring it might not be so on subsequent meetings. Try to not make a snap judgement, and keep looking interested. If you feel a topic has had enough of an airing, do try and gently change the subject, but only when the other person has had a chance to have his say.

Keep the tone of the conversation light. You are out to have fun, not to seek emotional support at this stage. That may come later if a relationship develops.

It is probably not a good idea in dating to talk about a previous relationship. You risk giving the message that you are not interested in this new person, and that all you really want is to be back with your former partner. How would you feel if the other person spent the evening talking about someone else? Being emotionally tied to an old relationship, or appearing to be tied, bodes disaster for a new one.

Humour always helps oil the social wheels – talk about amusing adventures you have had or of the funny situations you have been in. But don't overdo it and feel you have to be the entertainer of the date, or you may end up feeling under pressure. A sprinkling of humour with a genuine interest in the other person is a better balance.

Keep all early conversations to low risk level disclosures, and only hint at deeper issues (see Chapter 5). Your date will have to see you again to get to know the second instalment. Think of it as a little like Scheherazade, the narrator of *The Arabian Nights*, who started a story one night and left the end till the next – you can add a dash of mystery of your own.

Dating body language

When you enter a room you should look confident and have an upright posture. Give a big smile to the person you have arranged to meet so that you genuinely looked pleased to see him. Walk confidently but in a relaxed, easy manner. Take your time and don't bolt to the chair reserved for you, thinking that you will be less noticeable when you get there. Enjoy the attention of your date watching you as you approach.

Although you might think you come across as very interested by attentively chatting to the other person, you need to back that attention up with what your body is saying. As well as giving plenty of open smiles and eye contact, you also need to show that you find the other person attractive and get him attracted to you.

Preening also indicates attraction. For a woman, it includes playing with her hair by coiling it around a finger or selecting strands to slowly drag her fingers down, or flicking it back from her face, bringing beautiful hair to her date's notice. Sweeping hair back from her face to expose her neck is a gesture bound to bring attention to that delicate part of her body, especially if the exposed side of her neck is facing her date.

When men preen they might alter the position of their cuffs, touch their lapels or run their fingers through their hair. A brief raising of eyebrows at their date also indicates attraction. If this is combined with a smile, the effect is even more rewarding.

Ensure your body is angled towards the other person and that your feet also point towards your date (otherwise it looks as though you are poised ready to make your escape). Leaning forward shows interest as does mirroring what the other person does. For example, if she is sitting with legs crossed, so could you. Having your hands resting on the table in front of you helps to bring you closer and if the other person also has her hands on the table there is a much greater chance of having one of them briefly touched. Lightly touching the other person's arm or even hand, for brief moments, shows you like your date.

A word about physical intimacy – do take this at your own pace and don't feel pressured into giving too much too soon. Certainly on a first date, it's probably not a good idea to encourage too much intimacy. Once you feel comfortable with your partner, gradually increase the intimacy but at a slow pace so that you easily can pull back if you change your mind.

There are some people who remain wary of dating: for example, if they have been hurt in the past, have experienced rape or sexual abuse, or have come to an end of a long, monogamous relationship. In this case, they may feel so out of touch with dating and becoming physically close to someone new, that they want to take things very slowly. If this is how you feel, this is what you must do. Explain to your partner that you cannot yet contemplate a full physical relationship and explain why. If he loves you this should not be a problem.

What is attraction?

What makes you attracted to someone else? Is it physical appearance? Is it a feeling of like-mindedness? Is it is feeling that steadily grows from friendship and from doing the same things together? Is it related to how you think the other person would rate as a parent? Has it anything to do with the person's career prospects? Does age matter? Or do you take your romantic relationships very lightheartedly and consider the fun factor highest in your list of priorities?

It is very useful to have a good idea of what it is you are looking for before you go on a date.

Lucy

Lucy was shy and avoided extremely attractive men because she felt that they would not stay around long enough to get to know her properly since they had so many women eager to make their acquaintance. Lucy felt that they would not value her in the way that she longed to be valued. Concentrating on no more than average-looking men, Lucy found that when she got to know them and liked them, they became more and more physically attractive to her. Lucy's stratagem worked for her – she found a man she became very attracted to, was comfortable to be with and who took his time in getting to know her. He had the basic qualities she admired and that was all she could wish for.

You will need to decide the qualities that you admire in a person if you are looking for a lasting relationship. Just looking for someone that is physically attractive without other important attributes is not likely to make you happy. Although it may take time to establish whether these qualities are there, it will give you a foundation on which to build; and when you do find the right person the green light will be easily recognized. Good luck!

References and further reading

References

Howells, K. 'Social Relationships in Violent Offenders', in Duck, S. W. and Gilmore, R. (eds), *Personal Relationships 3: personal relationships in disorder*, Academic Press, London and New York, 1981.

Solano, C. H. and Koester, N. H. 'Loneliness and Communication Problems: subjective anxiety or objective skills?', *Personality and Social Psychology Bulletin*, vol. 15, 1989, pp. 126–33.

Vitkus, J. and Horowitz, L. M. 'Poor Social Performance of Lonely People: lacking skills or adopting a role?', *Journal of Personality and Social Psychology*, vol. 52, 1987, 1266–73.

Further reading

Argyle, M. and Henderson, M. *The Anatomy of Relationships*, Penguin Books, London, 1990 (previously William Heinemann, 1985 and Pelican Books, 1985).

Berent, J. with Lemley, M. *Beyond Shyness: how to conquer social anxieties*, Fireside (Simon & Schuster), New York, 1993.

Davidson, J. *The Complete Idiot's Guide to Assertiveness*, Alpha Books (Macmillan, Inc.), New York, 1997.

Duck, S. *Human Relationships*, 3rd edition, Sage Publications, London, 1998.

Fensterheim, H. and Baer, J. *Don't Say Yes when You Want to Say No*, Time Warner Paperbacks, London, 1991. (First published by Futura Publications, London, 1976.)

Gabor, D. *How to Start a Conversation and Make Friends*, Sheldon Press, London, 1985.

Glass, L. *Confident Conversation*, Piatkus, London, 1991.

Hartley, M. *The Assertiveness Handbook*, Sheldon Press, London, 2005.

Hauck, P. *How to Be Your Own Best Friend*, Sheldon Press, London, 1988.

Macaskill, A. *Heal the Hurt – How to Forgive and Move On*, Sheldon Press, London, 2002.

Nelson-Jones, R. *Human Relationship Skills*, Cassell, London, 1986, 1990.

Waines, A. *Making Relationships Work*, Sheldon Press, London, 2005.

Useful organizations

Addictions/substance use

ADFAM
Waterbridge House
32–36 Loman Street
London SE1 0EH
Tel: 020 7928 8898
Website: www.adfam.org.uk
(National charity for families and friends of drug users)

Alcohol Concern
Waterbridge House
32–36 Loman Street
London SE1 0EE
Tel: 020 7928 7377
Website: www.alcoholconcern.org.uk
(Produces a wide range of publications relating to alcohol use)

Alcoholics Anonymous
P O Box 1
Stonebow House
Stonebow
York YO1 7NJ
Tel: 01904 644 026
Website: www.alcoholics-anonymous.org.uk
(Supports anyone trying to overcome a serious drinking habit. Has online information and local contact details)

ASH (Action on Smoking and Health)
102 Clifton Street
London EC2A 4HW
Tel: 020 7739 5902
Website: www.ash.org.uk

(Provides information on all aspects of tobacco and campaigns to reduce the unnecessary addiction, disease and premature death caused by smoking)

Drinkline
Tel: 0800 917 8282 (9 a.m.–11 p.m., Monday to Friday)
(Offers information and self-help materials and support to drinkers, their families and their friends)

National Drugs Helpline
Tel: 0800 77 66 00
Website: www.talktofrank.com
(Gives free and confidential advice)

NHS National Smoking Helpline
Tel: 0800 169 0 169
(Helps smokers quit)

QUIT (The Stop Smoking Charity)
Ground Floor
211 Old Street
London EC1V 9NR
Tel: 020 7251 1551
Quitline: 0800 00 22 00
Website: www.quit.org.uk
(Helps people give up smoking and has educational resources)

Re-Solv (The Society for the Prevention of Solvent and Volatile Substance Abuse)
Helpline: 0808 800 2345
Website: www.re-solv.org
(Publishes booklets and videos about solvent and volatile substance abuse and can let you know of local agencies that can help)

Counselling and therapy

Anxiety Care
Cardinal Heenan Centre
326 High Road
Ilford

Essex IG1 1QP
Tel: 020 8262 8891/2
Helpline: 020 8478 3400
Website: www.anxietycare.org.uk
(Promotes the reality of anxiety disorders, obsessions and phobias and encourages those affected to use their strengths to work towards recovery and to maintain their recovery)

British Association for Counselling and Psychotherapy
BACP House
35–37 Albert Street
Rugby
Warwickshire CV21 2SG
Tel: 0870 443 5252
Website: www.bacp.co.uk
(Lists counsellors all over the UK, and gives information and advice)

The British Psychological Society
St Andrews House
48 Princess Road East
Leicester LE1 7DR
Tel: 0116 254 9568
Website: www.bps.org.uk/index.cfm
(If you want to consult a psychologist privately, they can send a list of chartered psychologists in your area)

Cruse Bereavement Care
Cruse House
126 Sheen Road
Richmond
Surrey TW9 1UR
Day by Day Helpline: 0870 167 1677
Website: www.crusebereavementcare.org.uk
(Offers help and counselling to the bereaved)

Eating Disorders Association
103 Prince of Wales Road
Norwich NR1 1DW
Tel: 01603 621 414
Helpline: 0845 634 1414

Website: www.edauk.com
(Information and support for sufferers of anorexia, bulimia and other eating disorders, and their families)

MIND (National Association for Mental Health)
15–19 Broadway
London E15 4BQ
Tel: 020 8519 2122
Mind*info*Line: 08457 660 163
Website: www.mind.org.uk
(Information service, books and pamphlets on many aspects of mental health)

National Phobics Society
Zion Community Resource Centre
339 Stretford Road
Hulme
Manchester M15 4ZY
Helpline: 0870 7700 456
Website: www.phobics-society.org.uk
(Information and support for people with phobias, anxiety, panic attacks and compulsive disorders)

Samaritans
The Upper Mill
Kingston Road
Ewell
Surrey KT17 2AF
Tel: 020 8394 8300
Helpline: 08457 90 90 90
Website: www.samaritans.org.uk
(24-hour help for people who feel suicidal or desperate for any reason – including loneliness, bullying, depression, suicide and sexual identity problems)

SANE
1st Floor, Cityside House
40 Adler Street
London E1 1EE
Tel: 020 7375 1002
Saneline: 0845 767 8000

Website: www.sane.org.uk
(Provides information and support to those experiencing mental health problems, and their families)

UK Council for Psychotherapists
167–169 Great Portland Street
London W1W 5PF
Tel: 020 7436 3002
Website: www.ukcp.org.uk
(Provides a list of local psychotherapists)

Racism

Commission for Racial Equality
St Dunstan's House
201–211 Borough High Street
London SE1 1GZ
Tel: 020 7939 0000
Website: www.cre.gov.uk
(Organization working against racism)

Institute of Race Relations
2–6 Leeke Street
London WC1X 9HS
Tel: 020 7837 0041/020 7833 2010
Website: www.irr.org.uk
(This organization is 'at the cutting edge of research and analysis that informs the struggle for racial justice in Britain and internationally')

Victim support and personal safety

Bully OnLine
Success Unlimited
P O Box 67
Didcot
Oxfordshire OX11 9YS
Tel: 01235 212286
Website: www.bullyonline.org

(Information available via website on all aspects of bullying including workplace bullying – see also 'Workplace Bullying' below – and discrimination at work on stress-related illness)

National Association for Support of Victims of Stalking
P O Box 1309
Kenilworth
Warwickshire CV8 2YJ
Tel: 01926 850 089
(Emotional support and advice for victims of stalking and their families. Provides initial advice on the telephone and further advice by correspondence. Short-term telephone counselling and referrals to local counsellors and therapists)

Rape Crisis Centre
Look in your telephone directory for details of your local branch.
Website: www.rapecrisis.org.uk
(Counsels victims of rape and sexual violence)

The Roofie Foundation
Monkswell House
Manse Lane
Knaresborough
North Yorkshire HG5 8NQ
Tel: 01723 367251
Helpline: 0800 783 2980
Website: www.roofie.org.uk
(Voluntary organization to raise awareness of the dangers of drug rape and to help and counsel victims. Date-rape drugs have the street name 'roofies')

The Suzy Lamplugh Trust
P O Box 17818
London SW14 8WW
Tel: 020 8876 0305
Website: www.suzylamplugh.org/home/index.shtml
(Charity concerned with all aspects of personal safety)

Victim Support
National Office
Cranmer House
39 Brixton Road
London SW9 6DZ
Tel: 020 7735 9166
Helpline: 0845 3030 900
Website: www.victimsupport.org
(Helps people affected by crime)

Women's Aid Federation
P O Box 391
Bristol BS99 7WS
Tel: 0117 944 4411
Helpline: 0808 2000 247
(Offers counselling, practical help and a refuge for women and children who are suffering any kind of harassment, abuse or violence)

Workplace Bullying
Website: www.workplacebullying.co.uk/links.html
(Information available via website)

Index